Conversations About Cancer

A PATIENT'S GUIDE TO INFORMED DECISION MAKING

Conversations About Cancer

A PATIENT'S GUIDE TO INFORMED DECISION MAKING

Michael Auerbach, MD

Chief, Hematology and Oncology
Franklin Square Hospital Center
Baltimore, Maryland

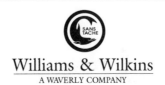

Williams & Wilkins
A WAVERLY COMPANY

BALTIMORE • PHILADELPHIA • LONDON • PARIS • BANGKOK
BUENOS AIRES • HONG KONG • MUNICH • SYDNEY • TOKYO • WROCLAW

1997

Editor: David Charles Retford
Managing Editor: Jennifer Eckhoff
Production Coordinator: Marette Magargle-Smith
Copy Editor: John J. Guardiano
Designer: Dan Pfisterer
Cover Designer: Tom Scheuerman
Typesetter: Peirce Graphic Services, Inc.
Printer: Vicks Litho

Accurate indications, adverse reactions and dosage schedules for drugs are provided in this book, but it is possible that they may change. The reader is urged to review the package information data of the manufacturers of the medications mentioned.

Printed in the United States of America

Library of Congress Cataloging-in-Publication Data

Auerbach, Michael.
    Conversations about cancers : a patient's guide to informed decision making / by Michael Auerbach.
      p. cm.
   ISBN 0-683-30072-5 (alk. paper)
   1. Cancer—Popular works.   I. Title.
  RC263.A93   1996
  616.99'4—dc20

                                           97-16212
                                             CIP

The publishers have made every effort to trace the copyright holders for borrowed material. If they have inadvertently overlooked any, they will be pleased to make the necessary arrangements at the first opportunity.

98 99 00
2 3 4 5 6 7 8 9 10

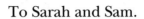

To Sarah and Sam.

Foreword

Most people fear cancer. This fear is magnified in the patient with cancer and his or her family. In part, this is due to lack of knowledge of the disease and the belief that, once one gets cancer, nothing can be done. In addition, many physicians, when talking to their patients have a difficult time informing them about cancer in words the patients can understand.

In this book *Conversations About Cancer: A Patients Guide to Informed Decision Making*, my colleague, Dr. Michael Auerbach, demonstrates that he understands the need to assist patients and their families in breaking through the barrier of technical language that often distances them from physicians and impedes their abilities to make informed decisions. In his book, he talks about specific diseases including discussions of screening, prevention, diagnosis, and treatment, as well as end-of-life decisions in terms that non-health care providers can comprehend. He provides the reader with concise, practical information that is easy to read. Hopefully, this should enable readers of this book to cope better when a cancer diagnosis is made.

Patients must realize that they and their families are not alone in their battles with cancer. Many different types of health care professionals will support them, but they themselves must become active, involved, and knowledgeable participants in their care. The ability to have clear, meaningful, two-way communication is a key element in permitting this to happen.

In pursuing this goal, Dr. Auerbach's book should be of help to patients with cancer and their families in two very important ways: first, by providing them with clear non-technical information that will help them understand the disease; and, second, by improving their abilities to communicate with health care providers and to share in any decision-making process regarding their cancer.

David S. Ettinger, MD
Professor of Oncology and Medicine
Associate Director for Clinical Affairs
Johns Hopkins Oncology Center
Baltimore, Maryland

Preface

A few years ago, just before I started writing this book, I was practicing golf on a driving range when a friend approached me. "Did you hear about Fred's wife?" he asked. "She has liver cancer. A surgeon told them he got most of it." My response was that cancer of the liver can sometimes be completely removed at surgery and in such cases is cured. He then asked whether it mattered that she had had breast cancer nine months earlier. I was shocked that this information could be so misleading. Breast cancer that has spread to the liver is a totally different disease with completely different management from cancer of the liver. I decided to write a book that would allow readers with a curiosity about or a personal interest in cancer to understand the viewpoint of an oncologist, a doctor who specializes in the treatment of cancer. In this book, I have tried to show how oncologists think about the individual diseases and how we approach them. I have tried to use language that can be understood by the lay public, and when forced to use words not commonly known by nonmedical readers, I define them parenthetically.

The book also discusses about how many of the treatments we use were developed. In explaining the way in which studies are done, the book attempts to negate the myth that participation in clinical investigations is tantamount to being a "guinea pig." The concept of randomization to different therapies or to therapy versus no therapy is explained. The discussion points out why using an unproven treatment can be worse than no treatment at all and why it is important to avoid the idea that "we have to do something" just because cancer is present.

More than anything else, the book is about communication between doctor and patient. It illustrates that it is not only essential, but also easier, for the physician, the patient, and their families when adequate time is taken to clarify what is being done and why. Within this explanation is the essence of empowering the patient to participate in the treatment decision-making process. The adage "You are the doctor and you know best" is condemned and is replaced by "These are the data" and "What do you think we should do?" This book explains carefully and meticulously how oncologists approach each of the diseases described in these chapters, what the dogma is about treatment, and where room exists for individualization of treatment.

Cancer is a common illness that frightens patients, their families, and friends. It still inappropriately carries the connotation of a death sentence and leaves patients feeling vulnerable and terrified. This book puts patients' expectations into perspective. In certain contexts, it discusses unfavorable outcomes plainly. In others, it stresses the optimism of curability and hopefulness.

My goal in writing this book was to create avenues for appropriate questions. If you have cancer, I hope you will understand what oncologists' goals are and what you can expect. If you are a family member or a friend of someone with cancer, I hope the book provides the information you need to understand the diagnosis and to assist you in your support of the patient's care and well-being.

Finally, the book provides a perspective on life ended by cancer. It talks about alleviating the suffering of the patient with terminal cancer and what I see as the physician-patient advocate responsibility for helping patients exit this world peacefully. The discussion centers on legal and available treatment modalities and stresses the observance of the patient's and family's wishes.

I hope that, after reading this book, you are more comfortable with the disease and, if that cannot be the case, that you have a better understanding of the many myths that belie optimum patient care and interaction among family, cancer patient, and oncologist.

Michael Auerbach
Baltimore, Maryland

Contents

Chapter 1

Introduction

No doubt, the diagnosis of cancer shatters most patients, their families, and friends. Most remarkable to me are how little communication occurs among many oncologists and patient and how little patients understand about their diseases. An initial visit in which all potential outcomes and available treatments are explained would avoid enormous heartache for both patients and physicians. The day when "You're the doctor and I'm in your hands" was the prevailing attitude is long past. Informed consent has become the standard of care. Unfortunately, because of the litigious nature of our practice, patients are required to sign meaningless, often legally worthless, pieces of paper filled with incomprehensible medical jargon. These consent forms sometimes are lengthened into tomes of patronizing sentences that describe every known side effect. Much of this paperwork could be eliminated if the physician were to sit down with patients and help them to understand potential outcomes and to participate in decision making about their own treatment.

PERSONAL BACKGROUND

Because I refer to myself in the first person, I would like to introduce myself to the reader. I am a hematologist and oncologist, a specialist in diseases of the blood and in the treatment of malignant diseases—cancer. I am about 45 years old and have been an oncologist for about 20 years. How did I choose my specialty? When I was a junior medical student in the early 1970s, I had a benevolent despot for a professor who was a hematologist. His skillful and scintillating teaching motivated me to enter his field. At the time, medical oncology was being born, and it was obvious that hematology, the only specialty actually to use chemotherapy, would be coupled with this burgeoning new field. Medical oncology was not part of my foreseeable future, and after a 3-year residency in internal medicine, which is required for entrance into oncology training, I decided to do subspeciality training in hematology. I began this training at New York's Columbia-Presbyterian Hospital, where the program already included medical oncology. Thus, by circumstance, I became a cancer specialist.

Most academic centers that train oncologists are involved in clinical investigation. To conduct extensive clinical studies in cancer, investigators must belong to a cooperative group, that is, an organization that pools data from many different places. In cancer treatment, such studies are referred to as protocols. I spend a fair amount of time defining protocols and describing them later in the book, but it was during my fellowship that I was introduced to clinical research in cancer treatment.

At the end of my clinical fellowship, I wanted a career in basic research in hematology (diseases of the blood and blood-forming tissues). I began my work in thrombosis (formation of blood clots) and hemostasis (arrest of bleeding) in the Columbia University Medical School's division of thrombosis research. I wish I had the constitution to have loved that type of work, but it was not for me. Patients were an almost nonexistent part of our work, and each month I seemed farther and farther from clinical medicine. After 2 years of pure laboratory research, I left to join the faculty of the Mt. Sinai School of Medicine in New York City, based at the Beth Israel Medical Center.

During my 5 years at Beth Israel, I was regularly involved in clinical research and did some public speaking at different medical centers. By a stroke of fortune, I was invited to Franklin Square Hospital Center in Baltimore, where I was offered the job of chief of the Section of Hematology and Oncology and director of the then nonexistent Cancer Center.

Franklin Square Hospital Center is located in northeastern Baltimore, and its catchment area (area served by an institution) includes many of Baltimore's heavy industrial plants. Cancer is a big business in this community, which has the highest incidence of the disease in the United States. The oncology department was not organized at this medical center when I arrived. The hospital wanted to be more closely involved in this clinically and economically important area. So, in an institution that had more admissions than any other hospital in Maryland, except the Johns Hopkins Hospital, I began to develop a comprehensive cancer program.

A comprehensive cancer program offers all aspects of cancer care. Surgeons who are trained to perform aggressive cancer surgery are essential for such a program. Radiation therapy must be available on site. Most important, the center must have a dedicated area for oncology patients that is staffed by specialized nurses. This last part is extremely important. Much of the therapy we offer is toxic. Most of the toxicity can be abated by appropriate intervention or prevention. Doctors are seldom around the hospital as much as nurses. When trained nursing is available at a specialized level, cancer care is vastly improved. Finally, because many cancers have no "best" treatment, new treatment protocols must be available. The availability of protocols requires participation in a cooperative group that conducts clinical research on cancer treatment.

None of the foregoing criteria were present at Franklin Square when I arrived. As my practice grew and as the possibility of a comprehensive cancer center became a reality, I was able to arrange for an area of the hospital to be designated for oncology. An attractive area was developed for treatment of cancer patients who did not need to be hospitalized.

I then had the hospital join the Middle Atlantic Oncology Program, a small, but active, cooperative group based in Washington, D.C. This connection gave us access to about 30 protocols for patients with a variety of different cancers and allowed us to become part of the multinational National Surgical Adjuvant Breast Program (NSABP).

Obviously, as people became aware that a community hospital in our part of town was participating in cancer research, my practice grew rapidly. With that growth, I

realized that part of our success was due to my willing-
ness to give my patients and their families relevant information about their cancer at the beginning of the
doctor-patient relationship. This practice not only is
valuable, it also is necessary. It became clearer to me that
most people afflicted with a malignant disease do not
have the chance to appreciate the process that leads to
decision making about their therapy. Patients seldom
understand why treatments and diagnostic tests are
done. A disparity often exists between the way cancer patients feel and the way "they are doing." Most of all, patients are rarely prepared for a bad outcome.

Some of what I say in this book is critical, but more
of it is explanatory. I begin by discussing a few general-
ities and then describe the major cancers and explain
how we approach their management.

DIAGNOSIS OF CANCER

Believe it or not, the diagnosis of cancer is better than
the diagnosis of a heart attack. Yet patients perceive the
opposite and have misconceptions about a cancer diagnosis that often worsen their performance through
their disease. "Performance" must be defined clearly. It
basically means how you are doing. Specific types of performance are referred to as performance statuses. They
are based on the degree to which one is able to move
around and stay out of bed, but those specific defini-
tions are not particularly relevant to this discussion.
When oncologists speak of good performance, we mean
that patients are basically doing well and can get around
and take care of themselves.

The term "cancer" is completely nonspecific. Our
bodies are made up of cells, and each organ has a
unique cell type. These cell types define the **type** of cancer, and it is essential to understanding of one's disease
to know the cell type. Few things upset or anger me
more than hearing a patient who has breast cancer that
has spread to the liver tell me that she has liver cancer.
This distinction may seem trivial to the nonmedical person, but both the management and the prognosis are

completely different in the two situations. This misunderstanding, which can have brutal consequences for families and patients, can be avoided by a 5-minute explanation.

How can people be expected to understand the difference between primary disease and metastatic disease if no one tells them? Do you know the difference? All tumors must come from somewhere. If cancer had no propensity to leave the site of origin, surgeons would almost always be able to remove the tumor and "cure" the patient. Cure means that the disease is gone, will not return, and will not require further therapy. I define cure and its unequal corollary, remission, later in this chapter. With regard to the cell of origin, breast cancer that spreads elsewhere is still breast cancer. The spread of a malignant tumor from a cell of origin (primary site) is referred to as a metastasis. Metastases can occur through the blood or the lymphatics, or they can even be direct extensions of a tumor by virtue of their own growth into adjacent organs. Nonetheless, metastatic disease has tremendous implications for prognosis because a metastatic tumor is rarely operable. The reason for the inoperability is that, once cancer spreads from its primary site, it usually does so in many different places, and to remove all the cancer cells is virtually impossible. Further, visible metastases are not usually the only ones present. In other words, even if a surgeon could remove all visible disease, new tumors would appear as part of the process of metastatic cancer. Rarely, a solitary metastasis occurs, and careful search for other sites of spread fails to reveal evidence of disease anywhere else. In this extremely unusual situation, surgical removal of the solitary metastasis can result in a surgical cure.

Why is this simple explanation of the difference between cancer confined to its organ (cell) of origin and a tumor that has metastasized so difficult for patients to understand and for doctors to explain? I am baffled by how little communication is used relative to this clear, important, and critical issue in cancer care. Once a definition of spread versus nonspread (metastatic versus nonmetastatic disease) has been made, appropriate treatment can be recommended. Often, more than one or two types of treatment are possible. Frequently, it is not clear which is the best type. Data on different treatment modalities usually are available and are not difficult to understand. Shouldn't patients and their families be involved in decision making?

PRINCIPLES OF CANCER TREATMENT

Unquestionably, radiology is our most potent diagnostic source. With the CT (computed tomography) scan and the even more sensitive MR (magnetic resonance) scan, entire sections of the body can be looked at without having to invade the body with a needle, scope, or blade. Ordinary x-rays (radiographs) still have great utility when we look at the lungs and bones, but the examination of body cavities has largely supplanted their use when we search for sites of metastatic spread. None of the tools is 100% accurate. Microscopic foci (points) of spread are routinely missed, and we have no reliable tool that lets us see microscopic disease.

Unfortunately, no blood test can tell us reliably whether cancer is present. This is not to say that blood tests that are useful in determining whether cancer may be present elsewhere in the body do not exist. However, the combination of all the tests tells us whether **evidence** of disease is present. The data can be gathered. When the data have been gathered, they should be presented to the patient in an understandable fashion. I believe that if a patient wants to have the data explained, and the physician is unwilling to provide the explanation, the patient should look elsewhere for care.

Let us assume that a cancer had been diagnosed somewhere in the body. Careful search for sites of spread fails to reveal any evidence of metastatic disease. The surgeon then says that the tumor should be removed surgically for cure. Certainly, that approach is correct for most cancers. What is not clear, however, is the unpredictability of removing all the disease. Most patients do not understand the difference between all disease and all visible disease. Therefore, a surgeon must let patients know that invisible disease can be present and missed. Only time provides that answer, but patients are entitled to understand the likelihood and, when possible, even the percentage of that likelihood occurring. For this reason, patients have follow-up care after surgery.

When a tumor is removed by a surgeon, and no visible evidence of residual disease is found after a careful search, is the surgery enough? Is it possible that microscopic foci of cancer exist somewhere in the body that could potentially be cured by chemotherapy if the chemotherapy were given promptly after surgery? For years, this concept of treating potentially present disease has been examined carefully in controlled studies. The name for such treatment is **adjuvant therapy,** which means the treatment of potential disease. The rationale for receiving chemotherapy or, for that matter, radiation therapy for disease that **may not** be there is difficult for some patients to understand. Yet, adjuvant therapy may significantly alter a patient's likelihood of suffering a relapse. For example, if a patient has a 30% chance of cancer recurrence after an operation, even after the surgeon has removed all visible tumor, treating the patient with chemotherapy could possibly decrease that 30% likelihood of recurrence to 15% or less. Indeed, such is the case for some tumors. The problem that patients seem to have with adjuvant treatment is the possibility that they already are cured by the surgery. Surgeons have this same problem. Why should they subject their patients to the toxicity of chemotherapy if these patients are cured or potentially cured? Here is why.

Most adjuvant therapy is well tolerated. Serious or life-threatening toxicity is extremely rare. Further, taking the chance of decreasing or even eliminating the possibility of recurrence of a tumor is worthwhile. Usually, when a tumor recurs (becomes metastatic), it is fatal. If, using the hypothetical example of the previous paragraph, you are one of the 15% of cancer patients who do not have a relapse, and it is **impossible** to know who will have a relapse, your life has been saved.

Unfortunately, patients never know whether adjuvant therapy mattered. For example, suppose a patient has a tumor removed by a surgeon and then receives adjuvant chemotherapy for 6 months. Forty years later, the patient dies of an unrelated problem. Did the adjuvant chemotherapy work? Would the patient have been cured without the chemotherapy anyway? In other words, was the surgery enough? Unfortunately, these questions are unanswerable. This concept is not difficult to explain before treatment is given, however, so patients undergoing adjuvant chemotherapy can resolve that they are undergoing treatment to increase their **chance** of being cured of an otherwise fatal disease. Not all cancers are affected by adjuvant treatment. Relaying the facts of such treatment before the commencement of therapy is beneficial for patients and their families.

How did the concept of adjuvant chemotherapy develop? As we discussed earlier, oncologists, in the infancy of our profession, thought that the use of chemotherapy after surgery to kill potentially present cancer cells could be useful. One does not simply treat patients on the premise that treatment may be useful, however. To determine whether a treatment works, carefully controlled, randomized trials must be done. In the case of adjuvant therapy, this adage is most important. The model for adjuvant therapy was developed in breast cancer. In chapter 4, I discuss in detail the way in which these trials are conducted and how the results are interpreted. For the purpose of this introduction, however, I just want to explain the basic concept.

Randomized Trials

Most patients are distressed by the idea that they may be randomized to receive no treatment. The standard question is: "If I need chemotherapy, what will happen if I am chosen not to get it?" This type of misunderstanding leads to a tremendous amount of lost data because many oncologists do not enroll patients in studies just to avoid such problems. For example, doctors who think patients may benefit from adjuvant therapy may simply wish to treat these patients **without any evidence that the treatment is beneficial.** Without clinical trials, we would never have learned that adjuvant chemother-apy **clearly** decreases the relapse rate in women with breast cancer who have cancerous (positive) lymph nodes under their arms.

What does all this mean? If a new treatment is avail-able for testing that has **not** been shown to be effective, patients should not feel slighted if they are randomly se-lected to not receive the treatment while participating in a study. On the other hand, however, if patients are cho-sen to receive the treatment, they should feel assured that it has been tested for appropriate safety. The efficacy of the treatment will be learned from participating in the study. Without such studies, or protocols as we call them, we would never learn whether certain treatments are worthwhile. This knowledge is extremely important in oncologic care because many treatments are toxic. If such a treatment will **not** benefit the patient, we should not offer it. Although this statement may seem obvious, the average individual would be surprised how often worthless treatments are administered because, "Well, they have cancer and we have to use *something.*" As I dis-cuss different types of cancer, this idea becomes much clearer. I also stress the importance of participation in co-operative group protocols (studies) whenever possible.

Let me take a hypothetical example to make the point. A surgeon removes a cancerous tumor itself and then takes a generous area of normal tissue around the tumor. The purpose of this procedure is to improve the chance of not missing local microscopic invasion into a surrounding area of tissue. (If that surrounding area of tissue is completely negative for any cancer after the pathologist examines the tissue under a microscope, that is referred to as "negative margins of resection.") The well-meaning surgeon tells the patient that all visi-ble tumor is gone. It does not matter what kind of tu-mor it was because we are talking hypothetically. All the radiologic tests done before the operation failed to show any evidence of cancer spread beyond the primary site. In other words, the patient had no evidence of metastatic disease before surgery, and the pathologist reports that the margins of resection were completely negative for tumor.

Considering the foregoing factors, the patient may well ask, "Well, it looks as if I'm cured, right?" The answer is "Maybe." The reason is easy to explain but often hard for patients to comprehend, or even harder to hear. After being removed, many cancers have a recurrence rate that is statistically predictable even without evidence of spread anywhere. Suppose I were to tell you that this hypothetical cancer recurs somewhere else in the body 30% of the time. We then ask, "Will the use of chemotherapy right after this surgery, which may have been curative, decrease that 30% recurrence rate to say, 15%? If the answer is yes, 15% of people who would otherwise die of this disease will not die of it. That number is important. However, how are we going to know? We cannot simply treat patients who want to be treated. We cannot blindly try an untested treatment. We need to enroll patients in protocols (studies). This is done by taking a patient with our hypothetical cancer and saying, "You will either be treated or not treated." This decision is made at random, usually by a computer, based on arbitrary factors such as a social security number. A decision is made whether a patient will be treated, and the physician follows the patient's course in exactly the same way with **or without** treatment. Usually, even treating physicians do not know whether their patients are receiving the drug. As years go by, oncologists look at the difference between the treated patients and the untreated patients.

A common reaction of many patients is to ask what happens if they are not treated. We often do not know whether a treatment works. The only way to find out is to conduct these randomized trials.

I am not trying to imply that patients with metastatic cancer should just be treated blindly without evidence that treatment is beneficial. Suppose a patient has a cancer that is not known to respond well to treatment. Blind, worthless treatment is toxic, expensive, and emotionally debilitating. The same principles about enrolling patients in carefully designed trials to look for benefit in treating potentially present disease apply in patients with metastatic disease. As I discuss the individual tumors that occur commonly in the United States and the developed world, individual studies are reviewed in more detail.

The findings of these studies teach oncologists to treat patients more effectively. These studies are done with wonderful cooperative treatment groups run by dedicated clinical investigators. The studies require the group effort of data managers, physicians, nurses, and statisticians. Studies such as the ones I discuss are available at university centers, at community teaching centers, and in private practice groups. The more patients enrolled in a study, the more we learn. Only 5% of potential study patients actually participate in protocols, however. At my center, every patient who is willing and able is placed in a study. Any patient not wanting to participate in the cooperative group trial is treated with the same enthusiasm and courtesy as a study patient.

Principles of Nonsurgical Treatment

I would like to end this introduction by describing the methods we use to treat cancer outside the operating room, that is, chemotherapy and radiation therapy. Conceptually, the goals of these treatments are not difficult. Cancer cells usually divide much faster than normal cells. As a result of their faster division, cancer cells have properties that make them structurally and functionally different from normal cells. Chemical reactions in the cancer cells often are different. All these differences provide the opportunity to attack the cancer cells **selectively** from the normal cells.

I do not suggest that chemotherapy and radiation therapy do not cause some damage to normal tissue. Obviously, these treatments are toxic. Unfortunately, that toxicity is often exaggerated. Oncologists usually are able to block many of the side effects, such as nausea and vomiting, which are the most unpleasant side effects, although they are not the most dangerous. Vomiting can lead to dehydration, which is potentially serious. Today, with newer and better drugs, most of nausea is obviated. Many chemotherapeutic drugs interfere with immunity and make the patient susceptible to serious infection.

We try to be alert to this susceptibility and stay ready to treat potential infections. Side effects are minimized with newer approaches to therapy. With these approaches, we can attack the cancer cells more vigorously with chemicals or radiation to **damage the cancer cells more than normal cells,** and to cause greater toxicity and cell death to the tumor than to normal tissue.

Two advances in the treatment of side effects have been so successful that they have revolutionized chemotherapy by allowing the use of much more effective doses of these anticancer drugs. The first advance is a drug for nausea called ondansetron (Zofran). I was skeptical about its use at first, but on trying it with drugs that routinely caused severe nausea, I was astounded by its effectiveness. The second drug, in a class of agents called "biologics," is made from a clone of a naturally occurring human product. It is granulocyte colony-stimulating factor (G-CSF). A granulocyte is a normal white cell that fights infection. By stimulating granulocyte colonies, G-CSF shortens the time that normal white cell counts are low during intensive chemotherapy. The use of this agent reduces the incidence of infection and allows oncologists to deliver much more effective doses of chemotherapy than otherwise possible.

Oncologists know the maximum tolerated doses for radiation and for all the chemotherapeutic drugs. We stay within these limits of tolerance and look for signs of early toxicity as we attack the tumor. Further, we measure the response with physical examinations of palpable tumors or with radiographs that show the tumor clearly. This principle of measuring disease allows oncologists to determine whether patients are benefiting. Individual tumors are known to respond to different drugs. When we know the drugs to use, we begin to administer them in the hope of shrinking the cancer while avoiding serious damage to healthy organs. The same principle applies to the use of radiation therapy.

When oncologists say that a tumor responds, we mean that, in studies already conducted, a particular disease has been seen to shrink or disappear with a specific type of treatment. The reason may be that the tumor has a sensitive chemical process uniquely inhibited by a drug or radiation, or a tumor may divide so fast that one can kill it by blocking its division without killing or blocking the division of normal cells. What is important is to understand that when oncologists use toxic drugs or radiation, we use them in a way that we know causes more damage to the cancer than to the healthy body. In doing this, we can shrink disease, prolong life, or improve the quality of life of someone with an otherwise fatal malignant disease.

Today, many cancers are curable with chemotherapy, even if they cannot be removed surgically. I define these tumors in subsequent chapters. I try hard not to exaggerate the successes of oncology and not to underestimate the toxicity of certain treatments. I am critical of some treatments used in the past, but I offer these criticisms only after I present the relevant data. If I am successful, my readers will be able to make intelligent decisions about available treatments, regardless of my opinions. Having learned about their individual diseases, cancer patients will be more qualified and better able to decide on treatment of their disease.

Chapter 2

Cancer of the Lung

FREQUENCY AND CAUSES

Lung cancer is the commonest cancer. Of all the cancers I treat, it also is the most frustrating. When I started medical school in 1972, lung cancer was the most common cancer in men and the third most common cancer in women. At that time, it was the second most common cancer in the developed world; cancer of the large intestine (colon and rectum) was the most common. Today, lung cancer has the dubious distinction of being the most common cancer in the developed world, the most common cancer in men, and the most common fatal cancer in women.* My frustration is worsened by the knowledge that approximately 90% of all lung cancer is completely preventable.

Lung cancer is one of the few diseases in which the cause has been unquestionably demonstrated. Oscar Auerbach (no relation to me), a pathologist at the Medical College of New Jersey, did research clearly demonstrating the pathologic steps by which cigarettes cause cancer of the lung. This research was hardly necessary because by all intents and standards, the statistical relationship between smoking and lung cancer was indisputable. Nonetheless, the tobacco industry has continued to argue that the relationship was circumstantial.

For my discussion, I assume that cigarettes cause lung cancer. More than 90% of patients with the disease have significant smoking histories. In the United States, however, we are beginning to see a decrease in the number of people who smoke and, more importantly, the number of people who start to smoke. Our government spends more than $300 million per year subsidizing a

*Breast cancer is more common but less often fatal.

crop responsible for one out of two acute-care hospitalizations in America. This same crop is responsible for lung cancer as well as many other cancers such as those of the throat, stomach, esophagus, mouth, and even bladder.

An enormous amount of publicity exists about the causal role of asbestos in lung cancer. Please do not confuse what I am about to say with other asbestos-related diseases, such as chronic disease in the lining of the lung or lung tissue itself, referred to as asbestosis. In addition, another rare cancer, called mesothelioma, is directly related to asbestos exposure. I am discussing the overwhelmingly more common cancer of the lung. Billions of dollars have been paid in workmen's compensation cases by asbestos companies to patients with lung cancer. Carefully controlled, meticulously done clinical research had failed to show a causal relationship between asbestos and cancer of the lung **in the absence of tobacco abuse.** Further, a synergistic effect of asbestos on tobacco abuse is minimal unless the asbestos exposure is massive. Nonetheless, the asbestos companies pay billions, and the cigarette manufacturers do not.

A remarkable article was published in June, 1989 by a researcher at the University of Vermont, Dr. Brooke Mossman. The article is the best review of asbestos-related disease I have ever read, but the end of the article leaves one with a bothersome thought. Small amounts of asbestos in buildings such as schools, terminals, and other public buildings pose no or virtually no health threat to the population. The United States is prepared to spend $150 billion on asbestos abatement. Asbestos is still the best insulator and fire retardant feasible for use in public buildings. Proper protection against asbestos exposure in workers should prevent asbestos-related disease. Asbestos abatement will not solve the major risk factor in lung disease—tobacco abuse.

By now, I am sure you've got my message. If you smoke, quit. If you don't, don't start. If you live with a family member who smokes, ask them to quit, and if you cannot, do the best you can to avoid the pathogenic air they exhale.

Virtually all lung cancer arises out of the lining of the

lung airway or glands in the lung. This disease is known as bronchogenic carcinoma. (The bronchus is the tube that brings air we breathe down into the lung. The suffix "genic" means arising from. Bronchogenic means arising out of the airway that brings air we breathe down into the lung.) Several types of bronchogenic carcinoma are known. What is important is to understand the approach to treatment of lung cancer and the way in which oncologists go about the decision-making process.

SMALL CELL CANCER

In my opinion, the first and most important categorization of the lung cancers is to separate what we call small cell cancer from the other types of lung cancers, collectively referred to as non-small cell cancer. The reason is clear and important. Small cell cancer of the lung, just one unique cancer cell type in which cells are particularly small and distinct, arises out of the airway lining and is virtually always multicentric in origin. ("Multicentric" means that where there is one, there is almost always more than one.) Studies on this cancer have shown that surgery is close to nonbeneficial and rarely if ever results in complete removal of the disease. Therefore, the debilitating effects of major surgery on small cell cancer of the lung should be avoided.

Small cell cancer of the lung makes up about 15 to 20% of all bronchogenic cancers. What is unique about small cell cancer is its exquisite sensitivity to both chemotherapy and radiation therapy. Therefore, when small cell cancer of the lung is diagnosed, medical oncologists commonly treat the patient. When such a patient is referred to me, my first job is to determine whether the cancer is confined to one lung, in which case it is called **limited-stage** disease, or whether it has spread beyond the one lung to both lungs or other organs such as the bones, the bone marrow, the liver, the adrenal glands, or the brain. This evaluation only requires a few simple scans, which can be done in any radiology department, and a bone marrow biopsy. This process is known as staging.

Bone marrow biopsy, discussed in more detail in Chapter 5, is a useful test for determining whether cancer has invaded the marrow portion of the bone. This test can be done in a hospital bed or in the oncologist's office. It is uncomfortable, but not extremely painful.

If small cell cancer is not seen on any of these tests, and if neither the radiologist nor the pathologist see any evidence of cancer beyond the lung, then the patient is advised that the small cell cancer appears to be confined to one lung and is what we call limited-stage small cell cancer of the lung. In this case, a vigorous program of **both** chemotherapy and radiation therapy is begun. The precise drugs and their method of administration are not relevant to this discussion, but the timing and intensity of the treatment are. This type of regimen is toxic and requires close monitoring. The patient must receive the treatment on time and at as close to full dose as possible. Further, if small cell cancer of the lung is untreated, the average survival is less than 3 months.

Oncologists generally agree on the type of chemotherapy given. Only a few different combinations are used today, all with similar effectiveness. All have similar toxicity, largely nausea and vomiting and bone marrow suppression. "Suppression" means to put down. Virtually all the drugs oncologists use "put down" the bone marrow and so cause the blood-forming organ of the body to decrease its production of normal blood. The major consequence of this suppression is infection because white blood cells, the blood cells that fight infection, are often decreased in number or eliminated for a short period. Fortunately, the amount of time the normal white cell count is low is predictable. A good oncologist knows this and monitors the patient closely when the white blood cell count is low. Often, prophylactic (preventive) antibiotics are used to ward off possible infections. Why do we take such a major risk? If we allow the tumor to grow during treatment, or to regrow after shrinkage, the battle is almost always lost, and death becomes inevitable. Therefore, oncologists and patients take the risk of a problem we can manage, such as infection, with intensive antibiotic treatment, rather than trying to handle a problem we cannot manage, recurrent tumor.

If a patient undergoing intensive chemotherapy develops a fever, oncologists can give antibiotics, which usually eliminate the source of the fever. When the patient's white count is low, however, this fever can represent a serious infection. The use of **granulocyte colony-stimulating factor** (**G-CSF**) can shorten the period during which the white cell count is low and can thereby decrease the likelihood of serious infection. However, G-CSF must be given by injection (patients can learn to inject themselves), and it is expensive. In the last several years, a class of antibiotics, the quinolones, has been developed. One of these, ciprofloxacin, is superior in preventing infections, specifically in patients with extremely low white cell counts. Giving the ciprofloxacin when the patients' white blood cell count becomes extremely low usually prevents the fever, precludes the need for hospitalization, and allows aggressive therapy against the cancer. Thus, many of the achievements in oncology are agents that allow the effective use of chemotherapeutic drugs. Nausea and vomiting have been drastically reduced by the wonderful drug ondansetron (Zofran). Without these agents, such aggressive treatment would not be possible.

Another major side effect of treatment is bleeding. The reason is suppression of the production of another normal cell, the platelet. The platelet, like the white blood cell, circulates with the blood and helps the clotting mechanism. Without platelets, bleeding usually occurs and can be severe. The role of the platelet in blood clotting is actually the reason that aspirin has become so important in the management of heart disease and stroke. Aspirin interferes with the action of platelets and makes them less likely to cause clots in vessels in the heart or the brain. This is still subject to great controversy, but the aspirin compound has sure become popular again as a result of it.

When we give these drugs, aspirin should be avoided, because aspirin interferes with the action of platelets. If platelets are low **quantitatively,** we should not give a drug that will make them abnormal **qualitatively.** With the avoidance of aspirin, the oncologist must monitor the patient's platelet count carefully and routinely. If the patient's platelet count becomes dangerously low, or if there is any sign of bleeding in a patient with a low platelet count, platelets should be transfused. Normally, platelet transfusions are available in any setting where oncology is practiced. Once again, oncologists and patients take the risk of a low platelet count because it is a manageable problem that may occur in an attempt to control the unmanageable problem of recurrent tumor or regrowth of tumor, in this case small cell cancer of the lung. The medical term for low platelet count is thrombocytopenia. ("Thrombocyte" means platelet; the suffix "penia" means decreased.)

Understanding the side effects, patients receive the appropriate chemotherapy. Usually, treatments are given every 3 to 4 weeks. During the administration of the drugs, oncologists monitor the tumor. If the tumor is in the lung, a chest radiograph may be used to measure it. The radiologist can determine the dimensions of the tumor, and one can then see whether the tumor shrinks or disappears. More often than not with this tumor, oncologists use the CT (computer tomography) scan of the lung. CT has become the workhorse of the radiology department and provides clear images of the body without invasion with needles, operations, or scopes. Most CT scans are easy to perform, readily available, and painless. Using our tool for measuring the tumor treated, oncologists can tell whether the tumor has shrunk or even disappeared.

Small cell cancer of the lung usually responds well to chemotherapy. The number of cycles, or complete treatments, given in this disease is six, and treatments usually last 18 to 24 weeks. The reason for six is not arbitrary. In the introduction, I discussed protocols or cooperative group studies. These studies on small cell cancer showed that fewer than six treatments gave too high a recurrence rate, and more than six treatments made no difference. Therefore, it is not necessary to expose patients to more toxicity with more than six cycles of chemotherapy because the controlled studies (protocols) showed that more than six cycles of treatment did not improve outcomes.

At the end of six treatments, our tool for measuring disease often shows that all the cancer is gone. As oncologists, we do everything we can to avoid the side effects of the treatment—antibiotics when necessary, platelet transfusions when necessary, and liberal use of drugs to prevent vomiting (antiemetics). Nonetheless, the small cell cancer of the lung will probably return. Therefore, after the chemotherapy is given, the oncologist asks the radiation oncologist to consolidate the treatment.

I use this term "consolidation," over and over again. It means to augment chemotherapeutic treatment right after it is given in an effort to destroy the cancer that we can no longer see with our tools such as the CT scan. In this case, the radiation oncologist administers a full dose of radiation therapy to the involved lung after, or in some cases during, the patients course of chemotherapy depending on the institution. Studies (protocols) have shown that this regimen decreases the chance of the cancer recurrence. However, radiation therapy also has toxicity. The skin can become irritated or even burned. Patients must be protected against this effect. Radiation also can cause bone marrow suppression, and blood counts have to be monitored closely, just as with chemotherapy. Every organ in the body has a maximum tolerated dose of radiation that it can handle without permanent and irreversible injury. Radiation is given in units called **rads,** or measurable amounts of radiation. The radiation oncologist knows just how many rads to administer to a patient's organ and does not exceed that dose, to preclude permanent damage.

When radiation to the lung is completed, one more therapy should be given—prophylactic radiation to the brain. The reason is that small cell cancer of the lung has a propensity to spread to the brain. When that happens, the disease becomes fatal. Studies have shown that, by giving prophylactic radiation to the brain, the incidence of relapse in the brain is significantly decreased. Once again, the radiation oncologist must continue to monitor the patient carefully for signs of toxicity.

With the foregoing treatment, 60 to 80% of patients will be completely free of disease by the conclusion of treatment. Unfortunately, more than 85% of these patients suffer a relapse by the end of the second year, however, and only 11–15% of patients survive for more than 2 years. Is it worth enduring this difficult treatment for a chance of 11% to live more than 2 years? **I cannot answer that question for you,** but I can explain it to you and let **you decide.** Once the patient understands the effects and side effects of treatment, as well as the goals of therapy, he or she can make the decision.

At the beginning of the discussion on small cell cancer, I mentioned **staging** the disease, or looking for sites of tumor spread (metastasis). These sites were the other lung, the bones, the bone marrow, the adrenal glands, the liver, or the brain. If the disease has spread to **any** of these sites, it is referred to as disseminated or extensive-stage disease. This disease is much more serious than limited-stage disease, and treatment is usually less intense because **cure** is virtually impossible. Numerous protocols at my institution and at others have examined different chemotherapeutic regimens for extensive stage small cell cancer. Radiation therapy is not discussed here because the disease is not curable, and **consolidation** has no meaningful role.

In extensive-stage disease, treatment is really palliative. "Palliative" is difficult to explain using the word soothing, because the treatment is toxic, with many side effects. Let us say you have a strep throat. You go to your doctor, who says you need penicillin. That is curative, because the penicillin kills the bacteria. In the meantime, however, your throat still hurts, and the doctor gives you an anesthetic spray to make your throat feel better. The throat spray is palliative. In the case of extensive-stage small cell cancer of the lung, chemotherapy is palliative. It shrinks tumor and thus often makes patients feel better. One-year survivals are uncommon; 2-year survivals are even less common, and the treatment is toxic. Patients are treated until they worsen. Patients and their families must understand this before embarking on a treatment plan.

Oncology has a long way to go before we can offer more hope for long-term survivals. New drugs will be necessary. (When these drugs are found, carefully designed protocols are going to be needed to learn how to administer them, to determine other effective drugs to use in combination with them, and the appropriate combined dose.) Small cell cancer of the lung rarely occurs without cigarette smoking. In 20 years of practice, I have not seen **one case in a non-smoker.** The disease probably is 100% preventable.

NON-SMALL CELL CANCERS

The other lung cancers, collectively called non-small cell cancer, are called that because their management is much different from that of small cell lung cancer. These non-small cell cancers are potentially curable by surgery. In the remainder of this chapter, I discuss how oncologists determine whether the cancer is curable. At this point, I need to define some terms. The first term is "operability," which means that the surgeon is able to open the patient's chest to see **whether the tumor can be removed.** Once the surgeon has access to the patient's chest and the tumor can be removed, the tumor is referred to as "resectable." Cure means that a tumor was removed or resected and did not come back. The only way to tell whether a tumor is cured is to wait, although oncologists have ways to predict whether a tumor will return.

How can a surgeon tell whether a tumor is operable? Tests and radiographs must be done first. One important criterion is the ability of the patient to tolerate surgery, especially given that at least a piece of lung and perhaps an entire lung will be removed. Because most patients with lung cancer also have chronic lung disease from cigarette smoking, the surgeon must determine whether a patient's breathing will be acceptable after the diseased portions of the lung are removed. Obviously, if a patient cannot breathe adequately after surgery, it makes little sense to perform a "curative" operation because the patient will not survive. Doctors determine respiratory ability by performing pulmonary function testing. It consists of a series of breathing tests with machines that can measure the amount of air moved when breathing and the size of the lungs before and after breathing. These tests can predict postoperative breathing capacity. If the prediction is that the patient will be able to breathe adequately after surgery, one hurdle in determining operability will be passed.

Another important question is whether the tumor has spread beyond the lung. This question is extremely important because removing the primary tumor, the lung cancer, cannot result in cure if the cancer has spread. Metastatic cancer may be present and can be missed by the best testing methods available. X-ray studies are usually obtained. A scan of the bones often is useful, especially if bone pain is present or if a blood test that shows inflammation of the bone is positive. A bone scan is easy to do, readily available, and completely safe. Some doctors order bone scans whether or not an indication exists, just to be safe. Other possible tests are a scan of the liver and a CT scan of the abdomen. An abdominal CT scan also allows examination of the adrenal glands, a common site of spread of lung cancer. If headaches are present or if the patient's behavior is unusual, a brain scan should be performed with either CT or the newer and more sensitive MR. These tools are usually available at most medical centers. If used judiciously, they can give useful information before to an operation for lung cancer. These tests may even prevent unnecessary surgery. If any of the foregoing scans are positive for tumor, the lung cancer should not be removed surgically, because such an operation offers no hope of cure.

Finally, lung cancers sometimes spread to the lining of the lung (pleura) and cause fluid to accumulate there. This fluid is referred to as an effusion. If a patient with lung cancer has a pleural effusion that contains cancer cells in the fluid, the tumor cannot be removed surgically, and an operation cannot cure the cancer.

The surgeon must determine by visualization whether a tumor can be removed. Much of this determination is not made until the patient's chest is actually open. Given that lung cancer kills 100% of patients if it is not surgically removed, the surgical risk is surely worth taking. The surgeon can inspect the patient's chest before surgery, using a scope to see around corners. This mediastinoscope is the same type of scope used to diagnose former President Reagan's colon cancer. The difference is that a colonoscope goes through the rectum, whereas a mediastinoscope is inserted into the chest through a small incision. The mediastinum is that area in the chest itself that is not the lungs, the heart, or the blood vessels to the lung and heart. In other words, the mediastinum is the remaining space. With the mediastinoscope, the surgeon can tell whether the tumor has reached an area in the chest that will make it impossible to remove. If all the tests for **operability** are negative (i.e., hopeful) the results of mediastinoscopy are negative, then the surgeon can attempt to resect the tumor.

The surgeon then must determine whether the patient has enough lung and airway (the tubes that carry air to the lung) **not involved by the cancer** to perform the surgery. For example, if the tumor involves the place where the trachea branches into both lungs, removal of the cancer will not be possible because the patient will be unable to breathe after the cancer is removed. That branch point or **bifurcation** of the trachea is called the carina, and involvement of the carina is a contraindication (condition that renders an action inappropriate) to resection. Involvement of the aorta, the biggest blood vessel out of the heart, also is a contraindication to resection. If no contraindications to resection are found, however, the surgeon then attempts to remove the last vestige of tumor, effecting a surgical cure. Nonetheless, more than 50% of patients who have resectable tumors develop evidence of cancer either in the chest or elsewhere and subsequently die of the disease. More than 50% of lung cancers are inoperable at their initial presentation. More than 50% of operable tumors are unresectable, and more than 50% of resectable tumors recur. Therefore, fewer than 10% of patients with lung cancer are cured of their disease by the surgeon.

Although options for patients with inoperable tumors are limited, radiation oncologists and medical oncologists offer many therapies to these patients. Radiation therapy can slow the local spread of the tumor, perhaps making the patient more comfortable. Research on this subject is controversial, but I believe that a palliative benefit exists. Chemotherapy was tried, and it failed until recently, when minor benefits have started to appear. However, lung cancer is the most common cancer in the developed world, and I cannot imagine our profession not treating it. Unfortunately, the medical treatment for this cancer has not been successful. At the 1988 American Society of Clinical Oncology* meeting, a summary of all of the protocols treating non-small cell lung cancer (remember that small cell cancer responds well to chemotherapy) was presented. No study showed a benefit in survival. With or without treatment, patients lived just as long. Some patients had responses and probably felt better as a result of having treatment, but overall, treatment did not prolong survival.

Therefore, newer and better therapies for this disease must be developed. The only way to make this happen is for oncologists to enroll patients in protocols using new treatments. Before new treatments become available in the medical community, they are extensively studied at investigative centers. Unfortunately, more than 95% of patients available for study are treated by medical oncologists who are not study participants. The reason is probably an unwillingness to participate in studies because of the extra work required. As chief of a hospital section of hematology and oncology, however, my office is managed, my secretary paid, and my billing done for me. Private medicine does not have such a luxury. Nonetheless, it can be done, and many private practitioners in the United States participate in clinical trials. In my opinion, until we find a treatment that is useful in non-small cell cancer of the lung, the cancer that makes up more than 75% of all lung cancer, we should not treat patients with toxic and expensive chemotherapy outside the framework of a study without telling them that treatment has not been shown to be effective. If patients understand this point, then it is reasonable to treat them. Many oncologists say, "I recommend that you take chemotherapy," without this type of explanation, however, and go ahead and treat patients. This practice is preventing the appropriate strides from being made with this disease.

---

*ASCO, our organization, has thousands of cancer specialists, as its members.

Chapter 3

Cancer of the Colon and Rectum

CAUSES, SCREENING, AND DIAGNOSIS

Cancer of the colon and rectum collectively can also be called cancer of the large intestine or large bowel. To summarize the digestive process, swallowed food travels through the esophagus, lands in the stomach, enters the long small intestine where much digestion occurs, and finally reaches the large intestines where the unused portion of food becomes stool. This last portion of the intestinal tract is what I discuss in this chapter.

The colon and rectum give rise to the second most common malignant tumor in the developed world, second only to cancer of the lung. In this chapter I try to define how we diagnose and treat this tumor. Before discussing the specifics of cancer of the colon and rectum, which from now on I refer to as cancer of the colon, however, I should mention that this topic is extremely controversial. Agreement on the best treatment for this cancer is by no means universal. Many therapies are recommended without adequate supportive data. Much of the reason for this controversy is a need on the part of the medical community to intervene in an otherwise difficult clinical situation. In setting forth what I believe to be the data as they exist, I attempt to be objective.

Think of the colon as a flexible tube with a center and a wall. The inside of the tube is termed the lumen, and it is the space in the bowel through which contents, such as stool, or feces, travel. The lining of the inside of the tube, called the endothelium, is made up of cells that are like little glands. These little glandular cells lining the inside of the tube of the large intestine are thought to give rise to cancer of the colon.

Imagine the thousands of pounds of food and liquid

that traverse our bowels in a lifetime. Each time something goes through the colon and into the toilet, it rubs against the endothelium. The actual cause of colon cancer, however, is still not known. No doubt, diet plays a role. In countries where carbohydrates such as flour and sugar are not refined, carcinoma of the colon is a rare disease. Nonetheless, we have been unable to prove that refined carbohydrate plays a causative role.

What appears to be more important is the transit of foodstuffs through the bowel itself. Foods or materials such as bran that increase bowel transit are believed to help prevent cancer of the colon. Conversely, materials that decrease bowel transit, or that increase the amount of time it takes for food to go from the mouth into the toilet predispose to cancer of the colon. The reason is not known, but it makes sense because slower-moving materials have the opportunity to sit against the endothelial cells for a longer period. Materials that are potentially carcinogenic will have the opportunity to be exposed to their target cells for longer periods. Nonetheless, this theory is still unproven.

Colon cancer received tremendous publicity when former President Reagan was found to have it. Using Reagan as an example provides a good opportunity to discuss how this disease is diagnosed. Medical adaptation of fiberoptic technology allows a physician at one end of the scope to pass a tube with a light and to see clearly at the other end. What is wonderful about the technique is that the clarity of sight continues around corners. A lens at the observer's end allows him or her to focus the light at the other end and to obtain a clear view of the lumen. A scope that allows the physician to see as far as the end of the rectum is called a proctoscope. A tube that allows the physician to go to the point at which the colon turns to go up to the left side of the body is called a sigmoidoscope. The tube that allows the physician to look at the entire colon, all the way to the right side of the body where the large intestine meets the small intestine, is called a colonoscope. These flexible scopes are much easier for patients to tolerate than the old rigid instruments and they provide an excellent means of examining the inside of the bowel wall.

In addition to scopes, radiographs also are available for looking at the inside of the intestine. By use of a liquid that x-rays cannot penetrate, such as barium, radiographs can help a radiologist to see masses in the colon. The procedure most commonly used to examine the large intestine is the barium enema. This tool is becoming less useful as fiberoptic colonoscopy becomes more widely available. Colonoscopy is becoming a standard test for individuals over the age of 50 years during **routine** physical examinations.

A good question to ask now is "When should a look at the inside of the bowel (by whatever means) be done?" A patient with any suggestion of bowel disease that could be caused by a tumor should have the colon examined. Symptoms that suggest a tumor include bleeding from the bowel and a significant change of bowel habits or stool character. For example, if someone who always has normal bowel movements suddenly develops thin stools, or if iron deficiency is present, an examination is in order. Blood contains iron, which is essential for normal blood function. When a red blood cell dies, as it normally does after circulating for about 100 days, the iron is picked up by a transport protein in the blood and delivered back to the bone marrow, where it can be used to make new blood. When someone bleeds, the iron is lost and needs to be replaced either in food or through iron tablets.

The only cause of iron deficiency in adults in the United States is bleeding. One reason is that even flour is fortified with iron, and it is almost impossible to become iron deficient by diet in the developed world without starving to death. We do lose about 0.5% of our iron each day in normal stool and sweat. Even if, in an extremely unlikely case, iron deficiency were due to dietary lack, the physician would need to ignore that possibility and assume that the cause is bleeding. One of the worst errors in medicine is the prescription of iron supplements without searching for a cause. If a menstruating woman has mild iron deficiency, the doctor does not have to obtain radiographs or perform a colonoscopy to search for a cause. If the cause of iron deficiency is not clear, however, it is **incumbent** on the treating physician to find the cause, or at least to try. Finally, it is becoming more accepted to perform a colonoscopy, or at least a flexible sigmoidoscopy, as part of a routine physical examination at the age of 50 or 55 years, and then at regular intervals thereafter.

When a mass is seen, either directly on the endothelium or as a polyp, a specimen must be removed for biopsy. That means that a tissue sample must be taken and sent to the pathologist for analysis. If the tumor is benign, it can be left in place or removed, depending on its size or the clinical situation. Some benign tumors can become malignant, and these should be removed before they actually become cancers. If the tumor is malignant, however, it must be removed, if possible, and a cancer operation needs to be performed.

Former President Reagan's colon cancer was found with a colonoscope. Fortunately for him, his cancer was confined to the colon and had not spread. The surgeon removed the cancer, and Reagan was cured. **Surgery is the only way to cure colon cancer.** If the colon cancer has metastasized, it can be treated with chemotherapy and the patient's life can be prolonged, as discussed in detail later in the chapter. Metastatic colon cancer cannot be cured, however. If the tumor is confined to the colon or its nearby structures, and the surgeon removes the last cancer cell, the tumor can be cured by surgery.

CLASSIFICATION

In 1932, a surgeon named Dukes used the degree of invasion of a cancer through the wall of the colon to classify the disease. Although the classification has been refined to some degree, this magnificent piece of work is still used to clarify cancers of the colon and rectum.

The Dukes' classification goes from Dukes' A, the least invasive or least severe, to Dukes' D, the worst type. A Dukes' A cancer of the colon is a cancer that involves only the inner aspect (endothelium) of the colon wall. That means that the tumor has not invaded the outer wall (serosa) or the muscle (which propels the stool through the intestine). Dukes' B cancer of the colon has invaded the outer wall, or muscle, or has even penetrated the serosa, but it has not spread to the colonic lymph nodes, which are small, glandular structures that filter materials from the blood. When the blood supply to the colon leaves the colon, it has the opportunity to be filtered by the lymph glands. Blood doesn't do this directly. A circulation of lymph vessels, called lymphatics, allows portions of the blood to go directly through the little lymph glands. (We have thousands of lymph glands in our body. If you have a sore throat and feel "swollen glands" in your neck, these are lymph nodes. If you have a urinary infection and feel swollen glands in your groin, these are lymph glands. Most importantly, cancers can spread to lymph glands before spreading to other organs. If the lymph glands are the only place that cancer has spread to, and the surgeon can remove all these lymph glands, the cancer is cured.) Colon cancer that has penetrated the wall of the colon and has involved the lymph nodes adjacent to the colon, but has not spread to other organs, is called Dukes' C cancer. This serious disease is potentially curable with surgery and possibly with adjuvant chemotherapy, which is chemotherapy for potential disease. Finally, colon cancer that has spread to distant organs such as the liver or lung is called Dukes' D colon cancer. This incurable and almost invariably fatal disease must be treated by chemotherapy, radiation therapy, or both, to gain some control of the disease or to prolong the patient's life.

The classification can be summarized as follows:

1. Dukes' A: colon cancer confined to the inner aspect of the bowel wall without invasion of the outer lining (serosa).

2. Dukes' B: colon cancer that has invaded or penetrated the muscle or serosa of the colon.

3. Dukes' C: colon cancer that has penetrated the bowel wall and has involved the lymph nodes adjacent to the colon.

4. Dukes' D: metastatic colon cancer.

APPROACHES TO TREATMENT

Obviously, the treatment of the disease depends on the type of cancer. Dukes' A cancer of the colon should be treated by surgery alone. More than 90% of patients with Dukes' A colon cancer should be cured by the operation. Unfortunately, Dukes' A cancer is not that common. The goal is to find the cancer as close to this stage as possible by performing routine, preventive examinations. Dukes' B colon cancer is also treated surgically. Actually, surgical procedures for Dukes' A and Dukes' B colon cancer are similar, and the surgeon rarely knows the difference until the pathologist has looked at the surgical specimen. The main difference between Dukes' A colon cancer and Dukes' B colon cancer is prognosis. Unlike Dukes' A colon cancer, in which most patients are cured with surgery, 20 to 35% of patients with Dukes' B cancer develop evidence of metastatic disease, usually in the liver, within 2 years of their operations. A 65 to 85% cure rate is still good, however, and no consensus exists about the use of **adjuvant chemotherapy** in Dukes' B colon cancer. Former President Reagan had Dukes' B colon cancer.

Dukes' C colon cancer usually recurs after surgery. Surgery is still the clear first choice for the disease. Nonetheless, 65 to 75% of patients develop metastatic disease, usually in the liver, within 2 years of surgery. Obviously, this figure is unacceptable because the majority of these patients will die of their disease. Adjuvant chemotherapy and radiation therapy have a major role in this type of colon cancer. The value of adjuvant chemotherapy for this disease became recognized in the late 1980s.

Many groups in the United States, including my own, have been investigating adjuvant chemotherapy in Dukes' C colon cancer by comparing treatment with no treatment in patients with the disease. This method may seem unfair to patients who are not treated, but we did not know then whether treatment made any difference, and if it did not, we would rather not have exposed patients to the toxicity of the treatment for nothing. It appears, however, that the use of chemotherapy postoperatively in patients with Dukes' C cancer of the colon, even though no visible or measurable disease is present, decreases the relapse rate. Data are still conflicting about how much chemotherapy to administer.

Metastatic cancer of the colon is not curable and is treated only by chemotherapy and radiation therapy. These treatments can shrink the disease, and even sometimes make it disappear, but the disease returns usually refractory (resistant) to further treatment. Not all patients with metastatic colon cancer respond to treatment, but those who do usually live longer than those who do not. For years, going back to the 1950s, even patients with colon cancer who responded to chemotherapy died in about the same time as patients who did not respond. This is not to say that patients who did respond, without any survival benefit, did not feel better or have much more useful lives. It simply states that, until recently, oncologists were unable to show a survival benefit by treating metastatic cancer of the colon.

One may ask, "Why then was it treated?" One oncologist on the faculty of Columbia University during my fellowship simply stated, "it's 40% of my business." This statement is unfair, however. Many patients did better with treatment. They just did not live longer. Study after study had negative results with colon cancer chemotherapy.

The drug that has been the mainstay of therapy in this disease is 5-fluorouracil (5-FU). This drug, which is given intravenously, interferes with cell division. Obviously, 5-FU interferes with normal cells as well, but it interferes with cancer cells more as do most chemotherapeutic drugs. The major toxicities of 5-FU affect the lining of the mouth, causing inflammation referred to as mucositis. Although mucositis hurts, is difficult to treat, and it usually resolves on cessation of the drug. Some patients develop diarrhea, but this is not common with standard dosing.

What is standard dosing? Until recently, it was the administration of 5-FU in a dose determined by body size (height and weight) over a 5-day period. Various means of administration have been studied. The drug has been given as a short intravenous injection called a bolus. It has also been given as a continuous intravenous drip called a continuous infusion. It has been administered into the liver, as well as directly into arteries. The drug has been given in combination with other drugs and at different doses. In these studies, some variability in the patients' responses were reported, but all these methods of administration had one thing in common: they did not prolong survival. Some were associated with better response rates than others, but survival was the same as no treatment at all.

In oncologic terms, **response rate** means that oncologists are able to measure at least a 50% decrease in the treated tumor. For instance, if colon cancer has spread to the liver, and the cancer is visible on an x-ray film, such as a CT scan, we measure the tumor before treating it and look for at least a 50% decrease in the measurable mass of the tumor. If this occurs, it is called a partial response or a partial remission. If all the tumor disappears, it is called a complete response or complete remission. In colon cancer, complete remissions were, and are, rare. If the tumor disappears forever, then the response is termed a cure. This does not occur with advanced cancer of the colon, regardless of the type of chemotherapy used, and it refers to metastatic disease, not to disease curable by surgery.

In these early studies, no matter what drug was considered, 5-FU had the most antitumor activity. The action of a drug can be altered by giving another drug that affects the way the drug is dealt with by the body, however. In addition, the drug can be administered in novel ways to alter the way it works in the body. In the late 1970s and early 1980s, two studies were begun at approximately the same time. Both have been published, and both treatments that arose from the studies are now used.

Two other compounds are available for altering the action of 5-FU. One of these compounds, PALA, alters the way in which 5-FU is used by the cancer cell and also by normal cells. Another drug is leucovorin, which is an expensive type of vitamin B. It alters the way 5-FU is taken up by the cells and increases the activity of the drug. Until recently, its only use was in conjunction with methotrexate, a drug used to treat lymphomas (cancer of the lymph glands; see Chap. 5). If high doses of methotrexate are given, fatal bone marrow failure can occur. Leucovorin predictably reverses that action and is used to protect patients receiving high doses of methotrexate. When it was learned that the combination of 5-FU and leucovorin had increased antitumor activity in cancer of the colon, the combination was studied widely.

In trials of the combination of 5-FU and leucovorin, an increased number of patients responded, as defined by demonstrable shrinkage of their tumors. However, none of the trials was able to show a survival advantage over the 5-day 5-FU treatment. Nonetheless, this new and much more expensive treatment received a tremendous amount of press. At about the same time, life-threatening toxicity—uncontrollable diarrhea—developed in some patients. Physicians using the combination of 5-FU and leucovorin had to watch closely for this side effect because it put their patients at risk of dying of dehydration.

At the 1987 meeting of the American Society of Clinical Oncology, the papers on 5-FU and leucovorin were presented at the plenary session, the well-attended and prestigious session at which the papers deemed most important are presented. Although many oncologists believed that the data are insufficient to be conclusive, the plenary session papers touted the superiority of the 5-FU–leucovorin combination over 5-FU alone.

At about the same time, the Middle Atlantic Oncology Program, the cooperative group to which I belong, completed its study on the use of 5-FU as a protracted infusion. A **protracted infusion** is administration of the drug, at a reduced dose, for 24 hours a day, by means of a portable pump and a permanently implanted catheter (a button in the chest wall to provide access to the veins). The treatment runs for 70 days at a time and stops at the end of 70 days for a 2 week rest period. The results of the study clearly showed an increased response rate, similar if not superior to the response rate with 5-FU and leucovorin in combination. Moreover, the protracted infusion is less toxic than the combination of 5-FU and leucovorin, and 5-FU is a much less expensive drug than leucovorin. Our well-received paper was presented at the 1988 American Society of Clinical Oncology meeting and was published in the *Journal of Clinical Oncology* the same year.

At the same meeting, a paper was presented by a Canadian group on a carefully controlled clinical trial of a comparison between the 5-FU alone and the combination of 5-FU and leucovorin. Different doses and schedules were compared. The carefully demonstrated conclusion was that there was no difference in the treatments in terms of survival. The report received little publicity, however. The 5-FU–leucovorin combination remains the mainstay of treatment of colon cancer in the United States.

As mentioned earlier, PALA alters the way in which 5-FU is used by the cancer cell. Our group, the Middle Atlantic Oncology Program, is looking at this agent in combination with our published program on 70-day protracted infusion. It is too early to tell whether PALA will add anything.

Dukes' C cancer of the colon, which has spread to the local lymph nodes but not to other organs, is potentially cured by the operation that led to its diagnosis, but it often recurs. When the disease recurs, it is incurable metastatic colon cancer. You may have read newspaper articles about the adjuvant treatment of this tumor by the combination of 5-FU and the antiparasitic agent levamisole. This study, done by the National Cancer Institute (NCI), compared the combination of 5-FU and levamisole with 5-FU alone and showed a modest, albeit measurable, decrease in recurrence over a 2 year period. As a result of the NCI data, these investigators advised oncologists that all patients with Dukes' C colon cancer should be treated with adjuvant chemotherapy.

When making treatment decisions, physicians are better sources of medical information than the popular press. 5-FU–leucovorin is a promising therapy. The best way to use it is not yet clear. Protracted infusion of 5-FU is also a promising therapy. The combination of this treatment plus leucovorin or PALA may prove to be superior. Patients need to know what the terms superior and useful mean, however. The advantage in terms of survival of either of these treatments is less than 6 months. Some dedicated clinical cancer investigators believe that there is no survival advantage, although some data show that chemotherapy may be useful and may even prolong life in patients who respond.

The NCI data on adjuvant chemotherapy for Dukes' C colon cancer have now shown a decreased relapse rate for patients with positive (cancerous) lymph nodes. Several groups are comparing different ways of giving the 5-FU–levamisole combination, and some groups have different therapies that include 5-FU. 5-FU–levamisole has become the standard of care for all patients with Dukes' C colon cancer.

In summary, for Dukes' A cancer of the colon, which is confined to the inner lining of the colon, the treatment is surgery alone. For Dukes' B cancer of the colon, the treatment is also surgery alone. No clear data support the use of adjuvant chemotherapy for cancer that has invaded the outer wall or serosa of the colon but has not invaded the lymph nodes around the colon itself. For Dukes' C cancer of the colon, which has spread through the outer wall of the colon and has invaded the local nymph nodes, surgery should still be performed, and adjuvant chemotherapy should be given. What type of adjuvant chemotherapy combination remains to be determined, but the 5-FU–levamisole combination is the current standard of care. Oncologists hope that one regimen will clearly prove to decrease the recurrence rate of this dangerous type of colon cancer. Finally, for Dukes' D colon cancer, chemotherapy and radiation therapy offer the only chance for managing the disease. Whether these treatments can prolong life is still not clear. Patients who respond to treatment have a slight prolongation of survival and almost certainly an improvement in the quality of life.

As a patient, you need to find a physician who will be honest about what you have to gain by one treatment modality or another. Then, make an intelligent decision.

Chapter 4

Cancer of the Breast

One out of 9 women will develop breast cancer over the course of her lifetime. This number is much higher than when I graduated from medical school in 1975. At that time, 1 out of 11 women was struck with this disease in her lifetime and even that number was rising from the 1950s and 1960s. Despite the near epidemic of breast cancer, the management of this disease is probably more controversial than that of any other tumor. Clear communication between patient and physician is of enormous importance in the management of this disease.

In no other area of oncology should the patient and her family be more involved in treatment decisions than with this illness. For years, surgeons have made most of the treatment decisions. When I was in medical school, it was common practice to perform a biopsy, obtain a frozen section for rapid diagnosis, and continue with definitive treatment without waking the patient up to consult with her. In fact, that was the standard of care. Fortunately, such is no longer the prevailing pattern of care. In Maryland, for example, a surgeon must wait 3 days from diagnosis to definitive treatment before operating, and all clinically appropriate treatment options must be offered to the patient before definitive surgery is performed.

My goal is to give the reader a reasonable understanding of the patient's role in decision making. To do this, the breast has to be defined anatomically, to explain the different kinds of cancers of the breast. I discuss risk factors and appropriate screening. Then I discuss diagnosis, staging, and treatment. I define how the results of this workup lead to an understanding of an individual's prognosis and, in knowing their prognosis, how patients are directly involved in making treatment decisions. I go into detail about surgery and chemotherapy and make clear when adjuvant therapy, which is the treatment of potential disease, is beneficial and when it is not. In breast cancer, adjuvant therapy is used to decrease the likelihood that the cancer will return after surgery. I discuss the different types of surgery and define each procedure. Finally, I review the newer ways to treat breast cancer both when it is confined to the breast and when it has become advanced.

RISK FACTORS

With the development of new assays for specific substances in the blood associated with the presence of breast cancer, discussing all the postulated risk factors would take a long time. What I think is important, however, is a discussion of the major risk factors and how a patient with these risk factors should be alert to the likelihood of developing the disease.

The most important risk factor for cancer of the breast is prior breast cancer. Women who have been treated for the disease and have no evidence of it anywhere in their bodies have the highest risk for cancer in the other breast. Fortunately, good follow-up care mandates regular breast examinations and regular mammography, as discussed later in this chapter. Sadly, I have heard physicians tell their patients that they are fine and no longer need follow-up care. Nothing could be further from the truth. One in nine women develops this disease regardless of risk, and prior breast cancer raises the number to one in six or one in five. After prior breast cancer, heredity plays the strongest role. What I mean by heredity is a mother or sister with breast cancer. To a small degree, the presence of the disease in a maternal grandmother is also a factor. This means that if a woman has a mother or sister who has had breast cancer, she should be alert to the increased likelihood (increased from one in nine) of developing the disease, and careful attention to early detection should be paid. Of course, the presence of this risk factor does not mean that it is more likely than not that the disease will occur. If we are going to attach any importance to screening for diseases, however, identifying a high-risk population is extremely important. Daughters and sisters of women who have had breast cancer are at high risk.

The remaining risk factors are less important, but they are associated with an increased incidence of cancer of the breast. Nulliparous (childless) women have a higher incidence of breast cancer than women with children. The risk of breast cancer in women who have had two children before the age of 25 years is decreased. Along the same line, women who have an early onset of menarche (menstruation) are more likely to develop breast cancer than women with late menarche. Similarly, women who experience menopause young are less likely to develop the disease than women who experience late menopause. What all this means is that female hormones play a role in this disease, especially estrogen. If estrogen stimulation is allowed to go unchecked, that is, early menarche, no pregnancies, and late menopause, breast cancer is more likely to occur than if the opposite is true: late menarche, lots of children at an early age, and early menopause.

These entities are the major risk factors. Other risk factors exist, but they are less clear and much less important. Nonetheless, the risk of breast cancer is one in nine for all women. If you have a risk factor, your risk is higher. Because this disease is often curable if caught early, intensifying our screening procedures for women at high risk seems to make sense. Judge for yourself.

SCREENING

Much has been said about **breast self-examination.** This simple procedure is useful, but it has been largely supplanted by routine **mammography** (radiography of the breast). Self-examination is still extremely important, however. If a woman notices a change in the skin of her breast, the structure of the nipple, or a new lump, she should have it evaluated by her physician. These signs are late findings, however. They are not always too late, but they are indeed much later than the early changes visible by mammography. The question is how often mammography should be done. Although no consensus exists, the following guidelines are generally accepted by the medical community: In a woman who has no major risk factor for breast cancer, the age for the first mammogram should be between 30 and 40 years. Obviously, if a woman has a major risk factor, this age should be lowered considerably, perhaps even to 25 years. The recommended frequency thereafter, at least until 50 years of age, varies from location to location but is usually every 1 to 2 years. Women over 50 years of age should have annual mammograms. With newer techniques, the radiation exposure is minimal, and the risk of radiation is minimal in comparison with the risk of missing early breast cancer. Still in all, 10 to 15% of breast cancers are missed by mammography. Therefore, in addition to breast self-examination, I recommend that whenever a woman visits her gynecologist, which should be annually, a breast examination should be performed.

DIAGNOSIS

Many different types of breast cancer are known. For the purpose of this discussion, however, breast cancer is considered a single disease, albeit one with diverse characteristics that change the approaches to treatment, monitoring, and evaluation. These characteristics of the disease also change the prognosis.

The breast is a series of ducts surrounded by fat. These ducts are used for the delivery of milk to the nipple when nursing, and the fat and other tissue make up the texture of the breast. By far the most common type of breast cancer begins inside the duct and is called **intraductal carcinoma** (cancer) of the breast.

When a breast mass is detected, either by feeling a lump in the breast or by mammography, which is much more sensitive than physical examination, a piece of tissue must be removed from that precise area and examined by a pathologist. This procedure, called a **biopsy,** usually is performed by a surgeon. If the lump can be felt easily, the surgeon does not need the help of x-ray equipment. If the lump cannot be felt, however, then a mammogram can localize the area and show the surgeon when the needle is in the right position. This lump or area can be diagnosed in several different ways, but, for now, let us just say that the area or lump is removed.

The pathologist then prepares the tissue for examination under a microscope. The first thing the pathologist tells the surgeon is whether cancer is present. If the tissue is all benign, management is complete, and the patient has no need for further tests or treatment. If the area is malignant, however, the pathologist must to tell the surgeon whether the malignant area, in this case a tumor, is confined to the duct or whether it has invaded or infiltrated the surrounding fat or breast tissue.

TREATMENT

If the tumor is confined to the duct, it is called **intraductal cancer** or **ductal carcinoma in situ.** If the tumor extends beyond the duct into the surrounding tissue, it is called **infiltrating or invasive intraductal carcinoma.** The difference in the management of these two presentations is tremendous. Disease confined to the duct is much less aggressive than disease that has invaded or infiltrated the surrounding tissue. Although important controversies exist about the management of both types of breast cancer, I explain the available treatment options and let the reader choose among them.

Intraductal Carcinoma In Situ

Let us start with the less aggressive of the two entities: intraductal cancer of the breast or intraductal carcinoma in situ is a cancer that has started in one of the ducts within the breast but is totally confined to the duct and has not invaded the surrounding tissues of the breast. This tumor is not aggressive, although it can become aggressive in rare circumstances. This ability forces us to treat the cancer as if it has the potential to kill, even though that potential is present in only a very small minority of circumstances. In other words, if you do nothing to pure intraductal cancer in situ of the breast, nothing more will happen in the majority of cases. That is a high risk to take, however, because if the cancer becomes aggressive, the patient can die. This possibility had led to the recommendation that a mastectomy be performed to cure this disease, as it almost always does. What I mean by **mastectomy** in this case is not the radical mastectomy most patients used to have for breast cancer. This operation, called a simple mastectomy, removes the breast, including the nipple, but leaves the underlying muscles of the chest wall and does not remove the lymph nodes under the arm (axillary lymph nodes). Even though the cure rate is 100%, and even though the operation is a simple mastectomy, the operation still removes the entire breast. Medical researchers compared mastectomy with removal of the lump, called a **lumpectomy.** Lumpectomy has the advantage of leaving most of the breast in place. This operation usually has superior cosmetic results and relieves many women of the devastating psychologic effects that can result from the loss of a breast. The result of that comparison were that mastectomy was better, but only minimally better. Therefore, the next step was to compare mastectomy with lumpectomy plus radiation to the breast. Radiation has the ability to kill cancer in the breast when it is given at the right dose by radiation oncologists, who specialize in the use of radiation to destroy cancer. After a lumpectomy, radiation to the breast can kill any remaining cancer cells. Obviously, given that researchers found that mastectomy was more effective than lumpectomy alone, some of the cancer cells in some patients must have been left behind. This was the reason for the next step in the study. The results of the next step were that lumpectomy plus radiation was as effective as mastectomy.

Despite these findings, however, lumpectomy plus radiation has not become the treatment of choice. Some surgeons do not explain these data to patients, and some others fail to offer patients any option except a mastectomy. In my opinion, it is wrong to deny patients with breast carcinoma in situ this information. In

Maryland, and in some other states, it is also against the law. Most surgeons, however, tell patients their options, and many patients elect to have the mastectomy anyway. Radiation therapy takes a long time, is expensive, and often leaves a shrunken breast.

The data need to be presented in a clear and understandable manner, so patients can make their own decision. With this disease, doctors cannot decide what a patient should do without informing her of all available options.

Infiltrating Breast Cancer

Carcinoma in situ of the breast obviously has an excellent prognosis. The tumor behaves in a nearly benign fashion when compared with invasive or infiltrating breast cancer. Invasive or infiltrating breast cancer has invaded the border of the duct in the breast and has spread into the surrounding breast tissue, which is usually the fat in the breast. This cancer has to be treated differently from carcinoma in situ, and much more information must be obtained by the patient because a cancer operation must be performed. What is a cancer operation? The answer is not simply a modified radical mastectomy. Over nearly three decades, the National Surgical Adjuvant Breast Program (NSABP) has carefully studied women with breast cancer who have received different treatments, to determine the best way to treat women with this disease. The NSABP is the largest such group in the world, and it has been a privilege and a pleasure for me to be part of this organization.

One of the most important studies performed by the NSABP is a comparison of the outcome of women with infiltrating or invasive breast cancer regardless of tumor size, axillary lymph node status (cancerous or not), or age, who underwent lumpectomy with axillary dissection (removal of axillary lymph nodes) with patients who underwent the older and more extensive surgery, modified radical mastectomy. The first part of the study showed that women with the more extensive surgery had a lower recurrence rate and longer disease-free survival (survival without cancer recurrence). Further, the rate of local recurrence (recurrence in the region where the surgery was performed) was higher in the women who received the lesser surgery. Clearly, the lesser surgery was not adequate. So, the NSABP then did another study to compare modified radical mastectomy (which includes removal of the axillary lymph nodes) with lumpectomy plus axillary dissection plus radiation to the breast. Thousands of women were studied. They were compared for overall survival and disease-free survival.

The curves are identical. This lack of difference held for tumor size, presence or absence of positive axillary lymph nodes, and age. This information was staggering, and it means that the modified radical mastectomy is equivalent to lumpectomy, axillary dissection, and radiation to the breast. It means that if a woman wants to preserve her breast and undergo breast irradiation, she can elect that course of treatment without concern that the lesser surgery is inadequate therapy. It also means that a surgeon who tells a woman that a radical mastectomy ensures that the surgeon "gets it all" is misrepresenting the facts, because data from the study are conclusive and are based on findings in thousands of cases. As oncologists, we have an obligation to make this point clear and to allow our patients to decide on their surgical treatment.

In uncommon situations, a modified radical mastectomy must be performed, such as when a surgeon is unable to close the breast in women with extremely small breasts. Extremely large tumors and tumors right behind the nipple should not be removed by lumpectomy alone. Otherwise, the two operations are equal, and a surgeon's personal preference should have nothing to do with which procedure the patient receives. Many women still choose the modified radical mastectomy. Lumpectomy, axillary dissection, and breast irradiation take much longer because radiation must be given over time, usually more than a month. Some patients are afraid (unnecessarily so) of radiation. Others simply want the breast removed. It doesn't matter why someone chooses a particular operation. What matters is that the **patient** chooses. Thousands of breasts are removed unnecessarily each year because surgeons have not explained the options clearly. As the public becomes more and more informed, however, unnecessary mastectomies will probably not be performed as often.

Chemotherapy

In 90 years of surgical experience with invasive breast cancer, the overall survival rates remain unchanged. The reason is unclear, but most oncologists believe that breast cancer is a systemic disease, which means an illness involves the entire body's ability to cope with a disorder. This hypothesis led to an enormous amount of research, which began about 35 years ago, to determine whether the use of the chemotherapy after surgery would decrease the recurrence rate of the tumor. This question is important because most women whose breast cancer recurs after surgery die of the disease. Even more unfortunately, this group of women comprises nearly 50% of patients with breast cancer.

Adjuvant therapy or adjuvant chemotherapy is used to treat **potential** disease. There is no disease to measure and no disease to follow-up. The treatment is given to alter the odds that the tumor will recur. The way adjuvant therapy was approached initially was to enter thousands of women into a study and randomly assign one group of patients to receive chemotherapy and the other group to not receive the chemotherapy. In doing this study, many different characteristics were determined about each patient and her disease, and careful and understandable statistics were kept. These careful statistics needed to be applied to each group of women, depending on the type of breast cancer. This categorization, based on prognosis, is called **stratification,** and each group of numbers about the benefit or lack of benefit of adjuvant therapy applies to its own specific group.

Stratification of Tumor Types

For the purposes of discussion, I assume that the breast cancer that was operated on showed no evidence of distant spread. That means that preoperative blood tests and radiographs showed no evidence of metastatic disease (disease that spread from the primary site). For example, the chest radiograph showed no disease in the lungs, and the bone scan showed no disease in the bones. After the surgery, the first stratification or grouping is determined by whether the axillary lymph nodes are involved with tumor. If they are involved with tumor, the disease is referred to as node positive, and if not, the disease is termed node negative. If the cancer is node positive, then the actual number of positive lymph nodes becomes important. For example, if the patient has no positive lymph nodes, the overall cure rate approaches 70%. That means that 70% of women with invasive breast cancer are cured if they have no positive axillary lymph nodes. If the patient has only one positive lymph node, that number goes down about 15%, to 55%, and if two lymph nodes are positive, the cure rate drops to 40%. As more and more lymph nodes are positive, the chances of recurrence increase. Most women who suffer a recurrence of breast cancer die of it.

The second stratification or grouping requires some explanation. The pathologist who examines the cancer after it is removed determines whether the tumor has or lacks **estrogen receptors.** The tumor itself is sent to the laboratory, and a test for the presence or absence of estrogen receptors is done. If these receptors are present, the tumor is said to be estrogen receptor positive, and if they are absent, the tumor is said to be estrogen receptor negative. Estrogen receptor positive is better because carefully controlled studies show that the recurrence rate is higher for tumors that are estrogen receptor negative.

So basically oncologists divide patients with invasive or infiltrating breast cancer into four groups. The first group is node negative, estrogen receptor positive (the group with the best prognosis). The second is node negative, estrogen receptor negative (the group with the second best prognosis). The third is node positive, estrogen receptor positive (the group with the third best prognosis). The fourth group is node positive, estrogen receptor negative (the group with the poorest prognosis). Tumor size also plays a role, but for the purpose of this discussion, it has little to do with treatment decision making.

The results of studies show that chemotherapy and hormonal therapy, alone or in combination, increase disease-free survival or overall survival in every group tested. This information is staggering because it can be interpreted to mean that all women with invasive breast cancer should be treated postoperatively regardless of tumor size, node status, or estrogen receptor status. Although this statement is not entirely accurate, it provides a charge to all physicians who treat breast cancer to make the facts clearly known to their patients. Just as with surgical treatment options, **patients must choose what they want to do,** with the help of their doctors.

Hormonal Therapy

I mentioned hormonal therapy previously. A medication called tamoxifen was invented shortly after the estrogen receptor was discovered. This drug has the ability to decrease breast cancer recurrence rates in women whose tumors are positive for estrogen receptors. This was learned by randomly assigning patients with invasive breast cancer positive for estrogen receptors either to a group that received tamoxifen or to a group that received a placebo. Results were that the tamoxifen-treated group had fewer cancer recurrences.

Before suggesting that the patients who did not receive tamoxifen were treated unfairly, remember that oncologists did not know whether tamoxifen worked at that time. And, it is always better to avoid taking a drug that does not work since all drugs have the potential to cause side-effects. In this case, tamoxifen improved the outlook by decreasing the overall cancer recurrence rate and increasing disease-free survival in all groups of women whose tumors were positive for the estrogen receptor.

Any surgeon who tells a patient after surgery that he or she "got it all" is misrepresenting the truth. Even a tiny tumor in a patient with negative axillary lymph nodes that is positive for the estrogen receptor has about a 10% chance of recurring. Those 10% of women with this tumor, who usually are told that their surgeon "got it all," die of their cancer. I now discuss each of the four groups (node positive and node negative and estrogen receptor positive and negative), the available treatments, and what should and should not be offered.

The first group, and the one with the best prognosis, is node negative receptor positive breast cancer. This has an especially good prognosis if the original tumor was less than 2 cm (a little less than an inch) in its widest diameter. With no additional therapy, these tumors are cured by surgery about 92% of the time. Because of this extremely high number, oncologists must be careful about offering additional therapy, especially toxic therapy such as chemotherapy. Tamoxifen, however, has little toxicity. To that end, the NSABP did a carefully controlled randomized trial in patients with primary invasive breast cancer that was node negative and estrogen receptor positive and compared tamoxifen alone with tamoxifen plus chemotherapy. The reason that no group received no treatment is that a prior study had demonstrated that tamoxifen was superior to no treatment.

The results of the study showed that the group receiving chemotherapy plus tamoxifen had longer disease-free survival and possibly even a higher overall survival. Within the group of patients, however, those with small tumors had no difference. In my practice, I explain these results carefully to my patients and tell them to choose what they want to do. I tell them that tamoxifen is probably good for them, but if they choose to do nothing, they are probably cured. I explain that, by intervening with either tamoxifen alone or tamoxifen plus chemotherapy, their likelihood of relapse may possibly be lower, but if they choose to take therapy, they will never know.

Are you confused by this last statement? It means that oncologists have no way of gauging whether or not the treatment mattered. Because 92% of the patients do not have a relapse, we cannot determine whether the treatment did anything if the patient has no recurrence. The only sure things are as follows:

1) If no treatment is taken and no relapse occurs, no treatment was necessary.

2)If treatment is taken and a relapse occurs, the treatment did not work.

If treatment is taken and many years later the patient dies in a car accident, without any cancer relapse, no one will ever know whether that treatment was necessary. Conversely, if no treatment is taken and the tumor returns, there is no way to tell whether the treatment would have prevented the relapse.

In this situation, the oncologist is an odds setter. Therefore, oncologists need to be detailed in offering treatment, when it is possible that such treatment may not be necessary. The majority of my patients with this type of breast cancer (node negative, receptor positive) refuse chemotherapy and take tamoxifen. Some are not sure and choose to enroll in the trial in which their treatment is selected at random, and a few choose to do nothing at all. The choice is theirs. The oncologist's job is to explain all options clearly.

Therapy for Node-Negative–Receptor-Negative Tumors

The second group comprises patients with node negative, receptor negative tumors. These tumors are more aggressive. Careful studies have shown that receptor negative tumors have a higher relapse rate when compared with receptor positive tumors. In the mid-1970s, the NS-ABP began comparing no treatment with chemotherapy in this group of patients. Chemotherapy clearly increased disease-free survival, and these data now show that overall survival also is increased. Most patients who experience disease recurrence die of breast cancer. Because of that conclusion, the NSABP appropriately performed another study comparing the chemotherapy regimen in the original trial with a more intensive regimen of chemotherapy. The result was that the more intensive chemotherapy regimen was better than the less intensive regimen. The name of the regimen that became the standard of care for this group of women is called CMF (C, cyclophosphamide; M, methotrexate; and F, 5-fluorouracil).

Because the study showed, after a carefully controlled

trial, that the CMF regimen was superior to the earlier regimen, the next study, which is ongoing, compares CMF with the more aggressive chemotherapy regimen we use in patients with positive lymph nodes. The purpose of this study is to determine whether an even more intensive regimen is better than the CMF regimen. The study then compares each group of patients: CMF versus the chemotherapy called AC, used in patients with node positive cancer (discussed later in this chapter), with and without tamoxifen. When the study is over, oncologists will be able to state which chemotherapy regimen is better and whether tamoxifen adds benefit to patients with receptor negative tumors as it does to patients with receptor positive tumors.

When a patient with breast cancer that is node negative and receptor negative comes into my office, I explain the data. I tell the patient that I recommend chemotherapy, but I do not know whether the more aggressive treatment is better than CMF. I also tell her that I do not know whether tamoxifen is useful in her specific type of breast cancer. I then tell her about the NSABP study and offer participation in the study. If the patient chooses to participate in the study, I treat her exactly as I would if there were no study, but I let the computer that randomizes the treatments in the study to pick the treatment. If the patient chooses not to participate, I recommend that she take CMF for about 6 months because **CMF is the treatment that has been proven best so far.** I do not offer the other treatments in the study because they have not been proven more effective than CMF.

Although I have stated this before, patients must understand what they are doing when they are receiving treatment, especially treatment associated with toxicity. Doctors must not prescribe possibly worthless treatments that have not been proven effective. In oncology, such carelessness must be avoided.

Treatment of Node-Positive Breast Cancer

Because node positive breast cancer has a worse prognosis than node negative breast cancer, both node positive–receptor positive and node positive–receptor negative cancers can be categorized as node positive. Earlier I used the term AC for the chemotherapy regimen used in node positive disease. The "A" stands for Adriamycin (doxorubicin) and the "C" for cyclophosphamide. Adriamycin is a more intense drug. It has more side effects and can only be used for a limited time because at higher doses it affects the heart irreversibly. The NSABP compared chemotherapy without Adriamycin with chemotherapy with Adriamycin in women with breast cancer and positive lymph nodes. The conclusion was that the Adriamycin-containing regimen was superior. Still, many of the women with positive lymph nodes who received the AC regimen suffered relapses. Therefore, the NSABP compared the AC with "A" plus more "C," to ask whether more was better. The answer is still pending. The NSABP is now comparing "more" with "much more." Once again, when women come into my office, I explain that they should take chemotherapy and why. I offer them AC, but I also offer them participation in the trial comparing the more intensive treatments. I explain that oncologists believe that more chemotherapy has a better chance of decreasing the incidence of relapse, but it has not yet been proven. If patients want to participate in the trial, I treat them exactly as I do if they elect not to participate, and, as before, I let the study computer pick their treatment. If patients do not want to participate in the trial, I offer them the current best regimen of AC known and treat them exactly the same way.

Much depends on a patient's age, her underlying health, the number of positive lymph nodes, and her ability to tolerate treatment. More intensive treatment is more toxic. With the development of newer drugs, however, the ability to control nausea has improved. Before the discovery of ondansetron (Zofran), the toxicity of these treatments would have been intolerable. Today, however, nausea and vomiting are often negligible, thanks to this marvelous compound. The ability to handle the effects of chemotherapy on the bone marrow also has improved with the development of drugs that protect or stimulate the bone marrow and of wonderful new and more powerful antibiotics. Chemotherapy is much better than it used to be when given intensively, and I know of no chemotherapy worse than recurrent cancer. Because most patients whose breast cancer recurs die of their disease, oncologists continue to look for better and better ways to treat this disease and to prevent recurrence.

Chemotherapy Before Surgery

I hope this discussion has made you think about breast cancer. I hope it has made clear that surgery is not the only answer to breast cancer and that agents such as tamoxifen and chemotherapeutic drugs can markedly alter the outcome of the disease. Given that surgery hardly alters the outcome of invasive breast cancer the first improvements in survival came with chemotherapy in addition to surgery, the NSABP and other groups are asking whether chemotherapy **before** surgery improves the outcome. Few patients are ever offered participation in this trial, because of physicians' referral patterns. A woman with a breast mass is sent to a surgeon, who rarely sends the patient to an oncologist before surgery. The current question is whether women who have breast cancer can improve survival if they receive chemotherapy before surgery. To enter this trial, biopsy of the tumor can only be done with a needle. Surgery of any kind before choosing the type of treatment is not allowed. Because most of my patients come to me after surgery or after the tumor is removed, they are ineligible for this trial. Patients who are eligible enter the study after the needle biopsy is positive for cancer. They then are asked to enroll in the trial with the careful explanation that we do not know whether preoperative chemotherapy is better than postoperative chemotherapy. We also select the chemotherapy used for patients with node positive cancer. If a patient is treated preoperatively, she may receive more chemotherapy than she needs. We believe that this risk is worth the benefit, but it **must** be explained carefully. If the patient still wants to participate, the computer in the study randomly selects the patient to receive chemotherapy first and then surgery or surgery first and then chemotherapy. In either event, the surgery and the chemotherapy are exactly the same as if the patient were part of the trial.

I have only about a dozen patients in this trial because surgeons did not often cooperate. Patients who received their chemotherapy before surgery have all done well and, to date, (about 2 years into the study), only one patient had a relapse, although that does not mean that more patients will not. This question is important because preoperative chemotherapy may become the standard of care, and such a trial is the only way to determine whether it is appropriate. With the study now closed, we are eagerly awaiting the final results.

As a patient, understanding your options will facilitate your experience with the treatment of breast cancer. It will make clear why things are done and will also allow you to play an integral role in the selection of your treatment. I only hope that this level of explanation becomes the standard, and that more oncologists participate in these valuable trials. All these trials contain treatments, and they compare the best known treatments with newer treatments that appear to be superior. Once the new treatments are shown to be superior, they become the new standard of care, and another step forward is taken toward successful management of this disease.

Bone Marrow Transplants

I close the chapter by a brief discussion of metastatic breast cancer. This illness is fatal, but oncologists are trying to delay the inevitable and possibly to cure a small subset of patients. Chemotherapy and hormonal therapy are the only ways to treat advanced disease. Many patients respond for a period before the disease becomes refractory (unresponsive) to treatment. When the disease becomes unresponsive, I try to control the patients symptoms and to make sure that the last period of life is as comfortable as possible. A small group of young patients with metastatic disease may be able to be cured with enormous doses of chemotherapy, however.

Unfortunately, these doses irreversibly destroy the bone marrow, and the patient is left without the ability to make blood—another fatal condition. Therefore, a new way to treat young patients with advanced disease is to harvest their bone marrow and to store it in a deep freezer, use extremely high doses of chemotherapy to eradicate the breast cancer, and give these patients back their stored bone marrow. Occasionally, this procedure results in a long, disease-free period, and some patients who have had bone marrow transplants are alive without evidence of disease. It is too soon to tell, but that is all we have at this time. We need new drugs for breast cancer. We need new ways to attack the tumor. As the search continues, we continue to look for new ways to treat the disease with the agents we currently have.

In summary, the best way to fight breast cancer is to learn your options. Make sure that your physicians take time to explain available treatments. If they don't, find another doctor. The art of oncology, especially in the treatment of cancer of the breast, is the ability to explain a patient's options to her. As oncologists, this is our moral and legal charge.

Chapter 5

Hematologic Malignancies: "The Liquid Tumors"

Up to this point in the book, the tumors I have discussed initiate in one of the organs in the body: the lung, colon, or breast. These tumors are referred to as solid tumors because the tissue of the organ is solid. The medical term for the tissue of solid organ is called parenchyma. Therefore, the tumors from the parenchyma or organs are called solid tumors. Tumors that come from the blood and the blood-forming and related elements, such as the bone marrow, spleen, and lymph nodes, are referred to as hematologic (heme, blood; -ogic, origin) tumors. Sometimes they are referred to as "liquid tumors." They are the leukemias and lymphomas. Several others are known but by far the most common are leukemias and lymphomas. Although many types of leukemia and lymphoma exist, I do not want to present an encyclopedic listing of these diseases. Rather, I want to explain how we approach them in a general way and how we oncologists approach our treatment plan. Few areas of oncology are more important because virtually all these diseases are curable, which means that treatment is stopped, it is no longer necessary, and the disease will not return. Some leukemias and lymphomas are more readily curable than others, but virtually all are curable at least some of the time. Therefore, the goal of this chapter is to provide a basic understanding of the diagnosis and treatment of these diseases.

In addition to leukemia and lymphoma, another common group of hematologic malignancies comprises the plasma cell dyscrasias (diseases that arise from the cell, which makes gammaglobulin, the plasma cell). The paragon of this group of diseases is multiple myeloma, which is discussed at the end of this chapter.

LEUKEMIA

My life has been influenced by leukemia more than by any other disease in medicine. I distinctly remember having a difficult time sleeping when I was 5 years old. My parents were out that evening, and my baby sitter left the radio on until I fell asleep. Suddenly, the show was interrupted with a news bulletin that the comedian Red Skelton's son had acute leukemia. The next morning, my parents found me reading about leukemia in *Compton's Encyclopedia*. Obviously, at 5 years of age, my comprehension was limited, so I asked by mother what leukemia was. Her reply, "cancer of the blood," stood in my mind for years. Mr. Skelton's son died in 6 weeks, and Mr. Skelton donated much of his fortune to leukemia research. Childhood acute leukemia was one of the first malignant diseases to be consistently cured. It served as a model for the development of chemotherapeutic regimens that now cure up to 40% of adults with acute leukemia.

The term leukemia means white blood cells circulating in the blood (leuk, white; -emia, blood circulation). This literal translation has been changed to mean malignant white cells circulating in the blood. White blood cells are made in the bone marrow. Of the many different types of white cells, only two apply to leukemia: the **lymphocyte** and the **neutrophil.** The lymphocyte is responsible for the production of antibodies, which are proteins responsible for helping our bodies to recognize foreign materials, such as bacteria and viruses, that are more easily destroyed by our immune system. The neutrophils, also called granulocytes, attack foreign materials such as bacteria and viruses. These cells are virtually essential for life because, in their absence, we are at the mercy of simple organisms that exist everywhere. For example, acquired immunodeficiency syndrome (AIDS) is a disease that impairs the immune system. Most patients with AIDS die of infections that usually do not attack people with normal immune systems.

Lymphocytes and neutrophils (or granulocytes) are produced in the bone marrow. Their parent cells, or cells of origin, are called **blasts.** The parent cell of the lymphocyte is the **lymphoblast,** and the parent cell of the neutrophil or granulocyte is the **myeloblast.** "Myelo" means marrow, and myeloblast is the name of the marrow precursor cell (parent cell) or the neutrophil. Leukemia occurs when the normal maturation of these cells is arrested and the parent cells, or blasts, grow in excess. During this growth, they replace the normal bone marrow and thereby destroy blood-making ability. Once the normal blood elements are too low to sustain normal function, death occurs rapidly. The average survival of a patient with untreated acute leukemia is about 6 weeks. Acute leukemia from the overgrowth of lymphoblasts is called **acute lymphoblastic leukemia** (ALL) and leukemia from overgrowth of the myeloblast is called **acute myeloblastic leukemia.**

ALL occurs much more frequently in children. It is more curable than acute myeloblastic leukemia, which is more frequent in adults. Many types of acute myeloblastic leukemia are all treated just about the same. Therefore, the important differentiation that must be made as soon as a leukemia is diagnosed is whether it is **lymphoblastic** or **non-lymphoblastic.** We usually refer to the acute myeloblastic leukemias as acute nonlymphoblastic leukemia (ANLL). I use the term ANLL for the rest of the chapter.

Chronic leukemia is the opposite of acute leukemia. The names of the chronic leukemias have the same derivations as those of the acute leukemias. The difference is that, with the chronic leukemias, the overgrowth is not the parent cell, or blast, but the mature completed cell. Therefore, an overgrowth of mature lymphocytes is called chronic lymphocytic leukemia, and an overgrowth of mature neutrophils or granulocytes is called chronic granulocytic leukemia or chronic myelocytic leukemia. The name does not matter. What matters is how oncologists make the diagnosis and what we do afterward.

Acute Leukemia

Although the treatment of ALL and ANLL is different, the principles are the same. The disease has to be eradicated or it rapidly regrows and kills. Treatment is with chemotherapy with drugs that can turn off the growth and division of the malignant cells so they die and do not return. Many drugs can do this, but these same drugs turn off the growth and division of normal cells as well. In turning off normal cell division, normal cells die. Therefore, our goal is to kill malignant cells or blasts, and allow the regrowth of normal cells so the blood can be repopulated with healthy and normally functioning cells. Fortunately, this happens when we treat acute leukemia.

The drugs that are able to perform this function are extremely toxic. The process takes nearly a month. During this period, a tremendous amount of support and care must be administered to patients with leukemia so they do not die while waiting for the normal cells to return.

Because the leukemic cells destroy normal blood production, the presenting signs and symptoms of acute leukemia are associated with a decrease in normal blood elements. If the decrease in normal white cells leads to an infection, the patient may initially have an infection, and the leukemia will be discovered when a blood test is done in the process of treating the infection. If the platelets are decreased, the patient may have signs of minor bleeding because platelets initiate the clotting process. If the red cells are decreased, the patient will have signs of anemia such as fatigue or malaise. A combination of these symptoms is possible. The symptoms lead the doctor to order a blood test, which usually shows the presence of leukemic cells, or blasts, in the circulating blood. Blasts should **never** be in the circulating blood. The presence of the blasts or of abnormal numbers of normal cells leads the oncologist to perform a bone marrow aspiration, which is necessary for the diagnosis of acute leukemia. Once the bone marrow shows acute leukemia, the oncologist must move aggressively and promptly.

The first step is to separate the disease into either ALL or ANLL. This distinction is easily made in the pathology laboratory using special stains that make it easier to see the abnormal cells. In a hospital accustomed to treating these diseases, results should be available in no more than 24 to 48 hours. While waiting for these results, oncologists and patients can make preparations for treatment that will require a month in the hospital and for the management of all the complications of having no blood production for nearly a month. The blood bank needs to be notified that special blood products will be needed. Many units of red blood cells and platelets will be transfused while waiting for the normal blood to return. Because white blood cells cannot be provided effectively, many antibiotics usually are necessary to help the patient through the period when he or she has no normal white cells. In my institution, I always ask a specialist in infectious diseases to assist in the management of the different antibiotics. The ability to provide the many support services in a skilled and efficient manner differentiates leukemia centers from institutions that do not and should not treat acute leukemia.

With intravenous chemotherapy, intravenous antibiotics, intravenous medications to prevent nausea and vomiting, intravenous fluids, intravenous blood products, and countless blood tests, a patient's arms can be turned into a pincushion. Access to the venous system to provide intravenous treatments becomes difficult. Further, the punctures become uncomfortable. Therefore, as soon as the patient is admitted to the hospital, we place a catheter near the patient's neck that goes into one of the large veins near the heart. This easy and safe procedure allows oncologists to have access to the patient's veins with two or three lines at a time. These catheters are called double- or triple-lumen catheters. The treatment of acute leukemia is nearly impossible without the use of such devices, which require handling by skilled staff.

The care of leukemic patients needs to be preemptive, which means anticipating problems and handling them before they become serious. Oncologists monitor patients' blood daily, examine patients several times each day, and pay special attention to their mouths, a frequent site of early signs of serious infection. Prophylaxis (prevention) is the order of the day.

If the treatment goes well, by 10 days to 3 weeks after

the completion of the chemotherapy, which usually lasts about 7 days, the bone marrow starts to be repopulated with healthy cells. This is preceded by a rise in normal cells demonstrable on routine blood tests. When this rise occurs, the bone marrow examination is repeated. If the precursors (parents) of normal cells are seen without an increase in leukemic cells (blasts), we know that the patient is going into a remission. If the bone marrow is filled with leukemic cells, a remission is not going to occur, and the patient is probably going to die soon. Chemotherapy can be repeated, but usually the first course of treatment is the one that works.

Overall, about 70% of patients with acute leukemia achieve remission during the initial chemotherapy. These patients are potentially curable. Unfortunately, if no further treatment is given, about 90% of these patients have a relapse within 1 year, and most of the remaining 10% have a relapse by the end of 2 years. Relapsed leukemia is almost always fatal. Therefore, the patient in remission requires treatment. This treatment is called **maintenance therapy.**

Maintenance therapy consolidates what the remission-induction chemotherapy accomplished. The difference is that, with maintenance treatment, the starting point is normal bone marrow, and the goal is to kill invisible leukemic cells known to be present. By doing this several times, oncologists can eliminate the remaining leukemic cells and can change the relapse rate of 90 to 100% to less than 50%. This maintenance therapy is not gentle. The chemotherapy is strong enough to destroy all the bone marrow cells, just as remission-induction chemotherapy did. Each time the bone marrow is destroyed, we must wait for it to grow back with normal cells, and during each waiting period, the same intensive supportive care must be given.

I feel proud of the job we have done in creating an excellent center for leukemia care at the community hospital where I work. We have started a program, now being offered in about a dozen leukemia centers around the United States, to see how best to treat patients with acute leukemia who are over the age of 50 years. Until recently, most effort has gone into the treatment of younger patients. Bone marrow transplantation is not a treatment. All it does is allow for the administration of huge doses of chemotherapy that destroys the bone marrow permanently. Bone marrow transplants rescue the dead marrow. The hope is that the chemotherapy that killed bone marrow to begin with destroyed all the leukemia at the same time. The problem with bone marrow transplants for leukemia is that elderly patients are unable to tolerate the period it takes for the marrow to graft (grow). They also are unable to tolerate the terrible toxicities that result from huge doses of chemotherapy. In our program, we compare the best-known intensive regimens for maintaining leukemic patients in remission that can be tolerated by elderly patients. By the time the study is complete, we hope to offer a higher chance of cure to patients over 50 years of age than ever before.

This treatment is intensive and toxic. Patients often die without going into remission. Most of those deaths cannot be prevented. Patients and their families need to be prepared, and they must know what to expect. This preparation removes anxiety and provides for much better acceptance of the untoward events that occur during this ordeal. For me, this is still the most exciting area of my clinical investigation, and I have always believed that the treatment of this aggressive and malignant disease is the most challenging and rewarding part of my work.

Chronic Myelocytic Leukemia

Chronic myelocytic leukemia (CML) is an overgrowth of normal white cells. Sometimes this growth becomes so intense that the blood actually becomes thick. Unlike ANLL, however, there is less urgency in the treatment of this disease. The problem with CML is that it **always** converts to acute leukemia. When this happens, the acute leukemia has a terrible prognosis. Therefore, the goal in management of CML is to prevent conversion to acute leukemia. To date, oncologists have not been very successful in achieving this goal.

The initial job of the oncologist with a patient with CML is to explain the treatment options. Unfortunately, most patients with this disease are elderly, so bone marrow transplantation is an unacceptable option. In younger patients with CML, however, a bone marrow transplant from an acceptable donor provides about a 40% chance of preventing recurrence. In older patients, several agents keep the white cell count low enough for healthy life. Agents such as interferon may prevent or delay the conversion to acute leukemia. Unfortunately, however, this event still occurs, and patients die of their disease—acute transformation of CML.

Chronic Lymphocytic Leukemia

Few diseases in hematology are less well understood by doctors outside the field than chronic lymphocytic leukemia (CLL). In my early years of medical school, I actually learned that this disease was almost always benign. Just like CML, CLL is an overgrowth of normal-appearing mature lymphocytes. The cells grow, and often high numbers are present in the blood. The high numbers often create alarm for both physician and patient, and the term leukemia strikes fear into the hearts of all patients who think they may have it. Unfortunately, CLL is badly named, as I will demonstrate.

This disease has five main presentations, called stages. The staging of CLL was done by my friend and colleague, Dr. Kanti Rai, director of the hematology and oncology program at Long Island Jewish Hospital in Long Island, New York and professor of medicine at the State University of New York at Stony Brook. His marvelous work with CLL has provided an understanding about who needs treatment, who will do well, and who will do poorly.

The first stage, stage 0 CLL, is nothing more than an increase in the number of mature lymphocytes in the blood. The rest of the blood is completely normal, the patient has no enlargement of the lymph nodes or the spleen, and basically, if the white count is not checked, neither the patient nor the doctor would ever know that stage 0 CLL is present. This condition is still called chronic lymphocytic **leukemia,** however, which sounds ominous. Stage 0 CLL should not be treated. It rarely progresses to a more aggressive stage. These patients simply need reassurance. Stage 1 CLL is the same as stage 0 CLL, except the lymph nodes are enlarged. Like stage 0, these patients do fine. The lymph nodes rarely are bothersome, and if they become so, they can be removed or treated gently. This stage of CLL rarely progresses, and patients do well without treatment, although they too need to be reassured.

The remaining stages of the disease, however, often require intervention. Stage 2 CLL is characterized by a high lymphocyte count with an enlarged liver or spleen, or both. This disease usually progresses to a fatal illness within 5 to 6 years. Treatment is tailored to minimize the complications of enlarged organs and to maintain adequate numbers of blood cells. Treatment does not alter the disease, however. Therefore, it should only be used to make patients more comfortable.

The same applies to stages 3 and 4 CLL. Stage 3 CLL occurs when the increased numbers of lymphocytes growing in the bone marrow cause patients' red blood cells to decrease and result in anemia, and stage 4 CLL is diagnosed when the increased number of lymphocytes growing in the marrow cause the patients' platelets to decrease. A low platelet count is called thrombocytopenia (thrombocyte, platelet; -penia, decreased in the blood). Treatment usually is indicated in stages 3 and 4 CLL, but it provides only temporary relief. We have made little progress in helping these patients, who usually die in less than 3 years. In the period that we are able to treat them (with drugs that do not alter the course of their disease), supportive care to maximize their comfort is in order.

The oncologist's important job with regard to CLL is to clarify the extent of the disease at diagnosis and to advise the patient what to expect. If the stage is one of the benign forms of the disease such as stage 0 or 1, patients should know that they do not need treatment, and the condition is leukemia in name only. If the stage is advanced, patients need to understand that treatment does not alter the outcome of their disease, but everything will be done to make them comfortable and functional for as long as possible. The adage and charge "never make the patient worse" is most appropriate here.

LYMPHOMA

A lymphoma is a cancer that arises out of the lymph glands. These glands, usually referred to as lymph nodes, discussed in other chapters, are all over the body. When you have a sore throat and develop swollen glands, it is the lymph nodes that are swollen. Lymphomas are suspected when these glands swell without other cause. They become enlarged, are usually nontender to touch, and are not associated with other medical problems.

With the treatment of lymphomas, hematology and oncology probably first came together. These tumors were the first to respond well to chemotherapy. If I am not mistaken, soldiers with enlarged lymph nodes who were exposed to mustard gas in World War I were noted to have shrinkage of their lymph nodes. Subsequently, nitrogen mustard became one of the first chemotherapeutic agents used to treat lymphomas. With the development of newer drugs and after years of clinical research with the lymphomas, these diseases have become models of curable cancer. Lymphomas are classified first by the pathologic type of the tumor (as determined by a pathologist) and secondly by the extent of disease in the body. The sites of lymphoma are important. Therefore, when a lymph node becomes enlarged and lymphoma is suspect, a surgeon removes the gland and sends it to the pathologist for microscopic examination. The pathologist's first and most important job is to decide whether the enlarged gland is malignant or just reactive. Reactive enlargement occurs secondary to a benign problem such as an infection. Malignant enlargement of the lymph nodes is not due to another problem, but rather to a growth of malignant cells within the node.

Once malignancy is determined, the first differentiation is whether the lymphoma is of the *Hodgkin's* variety or the *non-Hodgkin's* variety. Hodgkin's disease, a type of lymphoma, is associated with specific findings under the microscope and also with the presence of an unusual cell, the **Reed-Sternberg cell,** named after the doctors who discovered it. Once Hodgkin's disease is diagnosed, the oncologist must be aggressive in determining the sites of spread of the disease. This determination involves radiographs, computed tomography(CT) scans, nuclear medicine scans, and a bone marrow biopsy. It may rarely even involve an operation to examine the abdomen. This process is called **staging,** and it is important because Hodgkin's disease is usually curable. Even the most advanced Hodgkin's disease is curable in the majority of cases.

Four stages of Hodgkin's disease are recognized. In stage I, a single lymph node or group of nodes is involved. In stage II, more than one group of lymph nodes, for instance, the neck and armpit (axilla), are involved, but both groups are on the same side of the diaphragm. In stage III, more than one group of lymph nodes are involved, but on both sides of the diaphragm (the spleen is considered a lymph node for this purpose). In stage IV, tissues or organs other than lymph nodes such as the liver, lung, and bone marrow are involved. In addition to determining the stages of Hodgkin's disease from I to IV, oncologists also add the letter A or B, which refers to the presence or absence of associated symptoms. The symptoms are frequent fevers, major sweats, or loss of 15% or more of the body's weight. If any of these symptoms is present, the patient is said to have B disease, and if all symptoms are absent, the patient has A disease. Therefore, a patient who has no symptoms but who has involvement of the liver has stage IVA disease. A patient with symptoms and with involved lymph nodes in the chest and neck has stage IIB disease.

The reason that staging is so important is that treatment varies with each stage. If the stage is I or IIA, radiation alone cures nearly 90% of patients, and almost 100% if the disease is stage IA. If B symptoms are present, the cure rate with radiation alone decreases, and many oncologists believe that the presence of B symptoms means that chemotherapy is the treatment of choice. Patients with stages IIIB and IV, regardless of B symptoms, require chemotherapy. The treatment controversy arises over stage IIIA.

As stated earlier, stage IIIA Hodgkin's disease involves both sides of the diaphragm, lymph nodes and spleen only, and causes no symptoms. For radiation to cure stage IIIA disease, virtually all the lymph nodes of the patient's body need to be irradiated. The cure rate of about 70% with radiation alone leaves a 30% rate of relapse. This rate is high in such a curable cancer. The use of chemotherapy after radiation in patients who have a relapse, called **salvage chemotherapy,** however, cures more than half of these patients. The problem is that the combination of high doses of radiation and chemotherapy creates a high risk for a second malignant disease, especially leukemia. Patients with secondary malignant diseases usually have poor outcomes. Therefore, oncologists try our best to provide the least toxic treatment that is most likely to cure the patient the first time.

Because scans do not show definitely whether the abdomen is involved in Hodgkin's disease, I rarely recommend that patients with stage I or IIA disease undergo surgical removal of the spleen and biopsy of the liver or any suspicious nodes. This operation, called a **staging laparotomy,** confirms the stage of disease before treatment starts. This procedure can help to prevent unnecessary relapses. It seems like a lot to do just to pick one or two curative treatments, but the chemotherapy of Hodgkin's disease is intense and often causes sterility in men. Because most of these patients are young, this consideration is major.

The chemotherapy takes about 5 to 6 months to deliver. As with other hematologic malignancies, oncologists monitor patients closely for side effects and provide support such as antibiotics and sometimes blood products if necessary. With rare exceptions, however, patients tolerate their treatment and have no evidence of disease by the time treatment is completed. The same applies to those patients who receive radiation therapy. After the treatment is complete, patients are monitored closely for 2 years to look for signs of recurrence. If patients have recurrence at 2 years, the frequency of the visits can be decreased, and by 5 years, only an annual visit is required. Careful and meticulous care goes into the diagnosis and treatment of Hodgkin's disease to ensure that patients receive the best and safest treatment. The cure of advanced Hodgkin's disease is one of the most satisfying experiences a physician can have.

Non-Hodgkin's lymphoma is classified into three broad categories. The first category is **low-grade** lymphoma. These tumors do not require treatment unless they cause symptoms. Remember CLL (chronic lymphocytic leukemia) discussed earlier in this chapter; the same principle applies here. Treatment does not alter the outcome and only serves to relieve uncomfortable effects of the disease. These patients often live for years, even decades. Oncologists need to be circumspect in recommending therapy, which is toxic and can potentially make patients worse.

The second category of non-Hodgkin's lymphoma is **intermediate-grade** lymphoma. Depending on the type, up to 50% of these cancers can be cured with aggressive chemotherapy. The standard of care in the United States is to use a chemotherapeutic regimen called CHOP (cyclophosphamide, hydroxydaunomycin/doxornbicin, Oncovin, and prednisone). The chemotherapy is given every 3 weeks for six courses. Each course consists of 1 day of intravenous medication and 5 days of the oral medication, prednisone. At the end of treatment, the majority of patients are free of disease. They are then followed-up closely for signs of relapse. Patients who have no relapse at the end of 2 years usually are cured.

Unfortunately, unlike Hodgkin's disease, relapse of non-Hodgkin's lymphoma usually is fatal. Some patients can be "salvaged" with aggressive chemotherapy or a bone marrow transplant. This treatment is dangerous, however, and these patients, who are older than those with Hodgkin's disease, are less able to tolerate extremely aggressive treatment. Nonetheless, we often offer this aggressive approach to patients who so desire. I can think of no area in oncology where a clear and careful explanation of options is more important.

The last group of non-Hodgkin's lymphoma is **high-grade** lymphoma. These diseases are less curable, but they still are curable. Once again, intensive chemotherapy with CHOP is the standard of care, and the same applies with respect to post-treatment follow-up. Newer approaches with shorter, more aggressive chemotherapeutic regimens appear promising.

PLASMA CELL DYSCRASIAS

These uncommon diseases are not as well known as leukemia and lymphoma. Nonetheless, at any given time, I usually have about a dozen patients in my practice with plasma cell dyscrasias. Fortunately, most patients respond beautifully to treatment for an extended period. In addition, newer drugs are available for managing the serious complications of this disease.

The plasma cell comes from the cell in our blood-forming system that is responsible for the production of antibodies, which are proteins made by cells that are important in the immune system. The cells that make antibodies are plasma cells, which come from the lymphocytes. When the lymphocytes are stimulated to make antibodies, they become plasma cells and begin to produce proteins necessary for immunity.

Antibodies are necessary for life and have specific roles in preventing many diseases. When we get a vaccine, the purpose of the vaccine is to cause the production of an antibody that is specific against a certain disease. For example, when we are vaccinated against polio, the vaccine gives a message to our lymphocytes to transform into plasma cells and to produce an antibody against the polio virus. We make the antibody, and then when the virus enters our system, the antibody attacks the virus, binds to it, renders it ineffective, and allows its safe elimination.

Antibodies have different chains that make up their structure. Each antibody has two long chains (**heavy chains**) and two short chains (**light chains**). Many different variations of these chains allow for the antibodies to be effective at killing countless invaders of our system. The two major types of light chains are **kappa** and **lambda.** These chains can be identified by a readily available blood test. Because we have billions of these antibodies in our bodies, we have a relatively equal distribution of antibodies with kappa chains and those with lambda chains.

When a plasma cell dyscrasia develops, the abnormal plasma cell clone forms just one type of antibody, an abnormal antibody. Abnormal antibodies are identified by a blood test called electrophoresis and are characterized by the presence of just one type of light chain, either all kappa and all lambda. This abnormal antibody production is called **monoclonal antibody production** or **monoclonal gammopathy,** and it forms the basis of the diagnosis of plasma cell dyscrasia. It is basically the equivalent of an abnormal coin that always comes up just heads or just tails when flipped.

Not all plasma cell dyscrasias cause the malignant disease **multiple myeloma.** This disease is associated with destruction of bone, kidney failure, seriously elevated blood calcium levels, and elimination of normal bone marrow elements by the overgrowth of malignant plasma cells. The diagnosis of multiple myeloma is made by finding evidence of these disorders. When a monoclonal antibody is detected by electrophoresis, which oncologists order when a routine test shows high antibody levels in the blood, these characteristics of multiple myeloma are sought. The bone destruction is discovered by examining a series of x-ray studies called a bone survey, which consists of ordinary radiographs of the skeleton. Punched-out areas (**lytic lesions**) in the bones are diagnostic of multiple myeloma. Bone marrow aspiration is performed, and if the marrow is replaced by malignant plasma cells or if sheets of malignant plasma cells are present in the bone marrow, the diagnosis is multiple myeloma. This diagnosis can be made easily in the doctor's office within an hour of the patient's arrival. Kidney involvement is diagnosed by looking for light chains in the patient's urine. If a patient with a monoclonal antibody seen by electrophoresis has a monoclonal light chain in the urine, that disorder is called **light chain proteinuria** (protein in the urine). When light chain proteinuria is present in any significant amount in the patient's urine, most hematologists and oncologists agree that multiple myeloma is present and treat the patient appropriately.

On the other hand, if just the antibody is present in the blood as shown by electrophoresis, and if the patient has no destructive bone lesions, no involvement in the bone marrow, and no involvement of the kidney, the disorder is known as plasma cell dyscrasia of undetermined significance (PCDUS) or monoclonal gammopathy of undetermined significance (MGUS). This disorder is followed-up without treatment. It may convert to multiple myeloma in the future, or it may not. Such patients must be counseled carefully and must have their conditions explained with utmost clarity.

If multiple myeloma is present, however, treatment must be started. The purpose of the treatment is to prevent or to delay complications of multiple myeloma and to prolong the patient's life. Multiple myeloma is fatal either by bone marrow and bone destruction or by impairing immunity so that severe infections occur.

The time-honored therapy for multiple myeloma is the use of two drugs, melphalan and prednisone. Both drugs are taken orally. Although regimens differ, most oncologists administer the drugs monthly for about 4 or 5 days at a time. During treatment, the size of the monoclonal antibody in the blood or in the urine is measured, and a drop to a normal level is expected. Once this occurs, the patient is in remission, and a new decision has to be made. Either the drugs can be stopped, and the monoclonal protein in the blood can be measured on a regular basis with prompt resumption of treatment if the disease returns, or the biologic agent alpha interferon can be given in place of the drugs. The reason to stop treatment or to intervene with another agent is that multiple myeloma eventually becomes resistant to the melphalan and prednisone, at which time management becomes difficult, and intensive measures are necessary to keep patients comfortable before they die of this fatal malignant disease. Every month off the melphalan and prednisone is 1 month less for the disease to develop resistance to treatment. Alpha interferon clearly prolongs the "no treatment" period and, to that end, extends the patient's life.

Nonetheless, the average survival of this disease is less than 5 years. I bring this up because some information disseminated in the hematologic and oncologic literature and even in newspapers and journals has been misleading. This information revolves around intensive regimens of high doses of chemotherapy and even bone marrow transplantation for multiple myeloma. Although these regimens are able to cause greater reductions in the myeloma protein than the regimen of melphalan and prednisone, they have not increased survival or effected a cure. These regimens are usually toxic and expensive. At present multiple myeloma is not curable. Melphalan and prednisone are the standard of care. Anything else should be considered experimental.

In summary, progress made in the treatment of malignant hematologic diseases is among the best in all medicine. We still have a long way to go, but high rates of cure in patients with these types of cancer has served as a model for clinical research to achieve cures in patients with other malignant diseases.

Chapter 6

Testicular and Prostate Cancer

These two diseases are discussed together for several reasons. Both occur exclusively in men, and both are anatomically related, originating in the urogenital tract. Beyond these two similarities, however, these diseases are about as different as two cancers can be. Testicular cancer occurs almost exclusively in young men. In fact, although the disease is rare, testicular cancer is the most common malignant disease in men between the ages of 20 and 40 years. Testicular cancer is a rapidly growing high-grade malignant tumor arising from germ cells, and prostate cancer is a slow-growing cancer arising from the glands in the prostate. **Germ cells** are the cells that give rise to our sexual organs. These rapidly dividing cells produce rapidly growing cancers. As a result of these differences in cell growth, testicular cancers are among the most sensitive to chemotherapy and radiation therapy, and, when advanced, they probably are the most curable of all inoperable cancers.

Prostate cancer occurs almost exclusively in older men and is by far the commonest malignant disease in men over 60 years of age. Prostate gland cells grow slowly, and prostate cancer is usually a slow-growing, indolent malignant disease. Prostate cancer is either cured by surgical removal, or it is incurable.

In this chapter I discuss the screening, diagnosis, staging, approach to treatment, and prognosis of these totally different diseases with a common origin in the male urogenital tract. Important issues in decision making are carefully highlighted in an attempt to emphasize the patient's role in decision making. Because testicular cancer is so curable, the management of the disease is dogmatic. The patient must understand that accepting the oncologist's recommendations almost certainly results in cure. On the other hand, prostate cancer is a progressive malignant disease, and the effects of treatment must be clearly understood in deciding what course to take.

CANCER OF THE TESTES (TESTICLES)

Testicular cancer is rare. It occurs in 1 man in 50,000. Testicular cancer affects young men who are otherwise usually completely well. Therefore, in terms of lost years of life, it can be devastating. Testicular cancer also involves an organ that has an enormous emotional component attached to its loss. Therefore, men tend to ignore changes in the testicle. Finally, at any stage of disease, from a limited tumor to widely metastatic disease, testicular cancers are almost always completely curable.

Most testicular cancer is detected by finding a lump in the testicle. This usually occurs when the patient is examining himself or when a sexual partner is fondling his testicles. Less often, a physician feels a suspicious lump. Regardless of how the lump is detected, it must be evaluated by a urologist unless a physician is sure that it is a simple fluid-filled cyst. Such benign cysts, called **varicoceles** or **cystoceles,** are minor abnormalities and may not ever need treatment. If treatment is required, a simple urologic procedure can be performed to eliminate the problem. If the physician has even a remote thought that the lump or mass is solid, however, a urologist (physician specializing in the urogenital system) must be consulted because almost all solid masses of the testicle are malignant. Regular examination of the testicles is especially important in men who had an undescended testicle at birth. An undescended testicle, which stays in the abdominal cavity without descending into the scrotum before birth, is much more likely to develop cancer than a normally descended testicle.

If a urologist believes that a solid lump is present, the testicle must be explored surgically. Sticking a needle into the testicle to make a diagnosis of cancer is contraindicated. The procedure is dangerous, and it may seed cancer cells into one of the many vascular (blood and lymph) structures in the testis. Therefore, the urologist must make an incision in the patient's groin. This is called the inguinal approach. The testicle is then removed from the sac and examined. If a mass is present, the entire testicle must be removed, to permit a proper diagnosis and to ensure that no cancer is left behind. Sexual and reproductive function can be completely normal in men with one testicle.

Once the testicle is removed, it is sent to the pathologist, who examines it under a microscope. The pathologist then advises the urologist whether the tumor is malignant and, if so, what type of cancer is present. Testicular cancer is divided into two large categories: seminoma and nonseminoma. Seminomas arise from the cells responsible for sperm production. They tend to be much less aggressive and therefore require less intensive therapy. On the other hand, nonseminomas, of which several types are recognized, arise from the less mature cells of the testes, often consist of several different cell types, and require more aggressive management. Further, unlike almost all other cancers, nonseminomatous cancers of the testicle have blood markers that reliably predict their presence. These markers, beta human chorionic gonadotropin (hCG) and alpha fetoprotein (AFP), can easily be measured through a simple blood test. Most laboratories have test results in a couple of days. More is said about these two markers when I discuss the management of advanced nonseminomatous testicular cancer.

Seminomas

For the sake of this discussion, I assume that the pathologist is correct with a diagnosis of pure seminoma. At times, some question exists whether nonseminomatous elements are present in the cancer. In such a case, the entire tumor is assumed to be non-seminoma, and appropriate treatment follows, as described later in this chapter. I also assume that the markers, AFP and beta hCG, are negative for cancer. When they are positive for cancer, urologists treat the cancer as though it were nonseminoma, even though the pathologist's report gives seminoma as the diagnosis. At this point, the patient is ready to undergo staging procedures.

Staging is the workup performed with examinations, radiographs, or surgery to determine the extent of disease. In the case of seminoma, a good computed tomography (CT) scan of the abdomen and a chest radiograph are the only tests needed. If both are negative for cancer, two possibilities exist. The first is that these studies are indeed negative and the patient is cured. The second is that the CT scan of the abdomen is falsely negative, and invisible disease exists in the lymph nodes of the abdomen. It is virtually unheard of to find disease in the chest in patients with a negative abdominal scan, and therefore, a negative chest radiograph is adequate to conclude the absence of disease in the chest. Scans of bone and of the brain are not necessary because these areas are rarely involved with this tumor, especially in the absence of symptoms.

If the abdomen is free of cancer, then the patient will be cured with just the removal of the testicle. The medical term for the removal of the testicle is **orchiectomy.** A problem occurs when a patient has a false-negative CT scan of the abdomen. The cancer starts to grow. Because seminoma is so incredibly sensitive to radiation therapy and the cure rate is so high, oncologists do not subject the patient to surgery to examine the lymph nodes in the abdomen. We simply administer radiation therapy to the lymph nodes in the abdomen, where seminoma is known to spread. The patient is almost always cured. In the rare patient who suffers recurrence, the chemotherapy used to treat nonseminoma is almost always successful.

I have been practicing oncology for more than 15

years and have treated many patients with seminoma. I have never lost a single patient.

Nonseminomas

Nonseminomas (germ cell cancers of the testis) are divided into four types: teratocarcinoma, embryonal cell carcinoma, mixed terato- and embryonal carcinoma, and choriocarcinoma. Teratocarcinomas are interesting tumors because they arise out of tissue that is early in our development. Therefore, the cells of a teratocarcinoma or its benign counterpart, teratoma, can give rise to several different types of tissue, including hair or even teeth. The embryonal carcinomas and choriocarcinomas are more aggressive than the teratocarcinomas. The more embryonal elements in a tumor, the more aggressive is the approach to treatment.

Once the pathologist reports that the diagnosis is nonseminomatous cancer of the testicle, staging is begun. The reason that proper staging is so important is the extreme curability of this type of cancer, even after it has spread to the abdomen or the lung. One of the most important aspects of the staging is to repeat a test for the markers (AFP and beta hCG) after orchiectomy. These markers guide oncologists in determining the completeness of the patient's response to treatment. A CT scan of the abdomen is essential, as is a chest x-ray study. If the chest radiograph has even slightly suspicious findings, a CT scan of the chest should be done. Some oncologists (myself included) believe that a CT scan of the chest should be done anyway.

Markers Negative, CT Scan of Abdomen
and Chest Negative

A few years ago, oncologists would have not accepted this situation as one we could safely watch. Over several years, however, thanks to the superb pioneering work of Dr. Lawrence Einhorn at the University of Indiana School of Medicine, we have learned that many patients are cured with orchiectomy alone. This requires that we enter a period of careful "watchful waiting," in which the markers are measured monthly at first, and then several times a year for 2 years. In the first year, the CT scan is repeated at 6-month intervals. If the patient shows no evidence of disease for 1 year, however, markers alone can be tested for in the second year, and then only every 4 to 6 months for the balance of 5 years. If no evidence of cancer recurrence is found, then these patients with highly aggressive cancer of the testicle have been cured by orchiectomy alone.

If the markers start to rise, or if the CT scan becomes positive for cancer, however, the patient must receive chemotherapy to prevent the cancer from spreading. This disease is highly aggressive and fatal if untreated. The chemotherapy for this disease has all been developed since the 1970s.

Markers Positive, CT Scan of the Abdomen and Chest Negative

This situation is much more worrisome. It suggests that the CT scan is falsely negative and residual disease is left behind. In this circumstance, two options exist. Oncologists can treat the patient with two brief cycles of chemotherapy using cisplatinum, bleomycin, and etoposide, or we can ask a urologist to perform a major operation and remove the lymph nodes in the abdomen. This procedure can leave a patient sterile, impotent, or both. Fortunately, newer techniques, called **nerve-sparing surgery,** have decreased the incidence of these side effects. After either treatment is selected, the patient must be followed-up with the same close "watchful waiting" as in staging for patients with negative markers and test results. What would you chose? In either event, the disease is curable. Because of this extreme curability, some oncologists even advocate careful follow-up of the patient to see whether the markers disappear. This approach is reasonable provided continuity exists between patient and oncologist. Some patients are emotionally unable to tolerate watchful waiting and require treatment. Others are perfectly comfortable waiting to see what happens. Few areas in my field require better communication between doctor and patient.

CT Scan of the Abdomen or Chest Positive

Because disease is left behind after orchiectomy, the only question in patients with this stage of testicular cancer is how to treat. If the only positive area is the abdomen, the patient has the option to undergo surgery without chemotherapy and be followed-up closely for cancer recurrence. Another option is to undergo chemotherapy without surgery and be followed-up closely for cancer recurrence. The amount of chemotherapy used is based on the amount of disease, but the real decision is between three and four cycles of treatment. Treatment takes about 5 days in the hospital and used to be nauseating. With the wonderful new drug, ondansetron, for nausea and vomiting, however, treatment is tolerated beautifully and, with the exception of being in the hospital for nearly a week, is benign. The treatment is repeated every 3 weeks for three or four cycles, and at the completion of the chemotherapy, the CT scans and the marker measurements are repeated. Virtually every patient is cured.

Testicular cancer is the model for curable cancer. Careful clinical trials using more and more active drugs have led us to conquer this killer of young men. It is probably the only disease in oncology, with the possible exception of Hodgkin's disease (see Chap. 5) in which investigators have actually compared curable therapy with less therapy in an attempt to decrease the amount of chemotherapy given. It was only possible to do this because the cure rate is so high even if initial therapy fails.

The oncologist must tell the patient what is going to take place. Then treatment should be started smoothly, and problems and contingencies dealt with promptly. The cure of advanced testicular cancer is among the most gratifying moments in my work. As with semi-

noma, I have never lost a patient with nonseminomatous cancer of the testicle, regardless of how advanced
the disease.

CANCER OF THE PROSTATE GLAND

As hopeful as the treatment of advanced testicular cancer is, the treatment of advanced prostate cancer is
hopeless. Therefore, early detection of this disease is
most important. Cancer of the prostate is the most common cancer in men over 60 years of age. With the one
exception of cancer of the lung, prostate cancer is the
leading cause of cancer-related death in men. The
American Cancer Society estimates that more than
110,000 cases of prostate cancer are diagnosed annually. Of those diagnosed, 30,000 patients die as a direct
result of the disease.

The real problem with prostate cancer is that it is
virtually asymptomatic in its early stages. Further, the most
common symptom of early prostate cancer is difficulty in
urinating or a change in the character of the stream during urination. These symptoms are commonly caused by
other conditions involving the prostate such as inflammation, infection, or benign enlargement of the gland itself. This last condition, **benign prostatic hypertrophy,** occurs in almost all men, depending on their age. What this
really means is that it is too late to wait for the disease to
become obvious. Physicians must screen patients for
prostate cancer. Although prostate cancer can metastasize to other organs of the body, it is a slow-growing tumor,
and complacency can lead to a false sense of security.

The prostate gland is a walnut-sized gland located
between the urinary bladder and the urethra. The urethra is the tube that carries urine from the bladder
through the penis to the outside of the body. Because
the prostate gland sits between the bladder and the urethra, it forms a small portion of the urinary channel.
The main function of the prostate is as a sexual organ,
however. The prostate produces a large portion of the
fluid comprising the semen. The gland is not essential

for life, but it is essential for fertility, and impotence often occurs in its absence. As the gland enlarges, for any reason, it compromises the urination. This condition may cause pain, but usually the first symptom is a decrease in the strength of the urine stream.

Patients complain that they are having trouble urinating. When that occurs, a urologist usually is consulted. An infection of the prostate is diagnosed, the gland is found to be enlarged, or a tumor of the prostate is felt. Waiting for symptoms to occur is inefficient and dangerous. Therefore, all men over 50 years of age, the age group in which more than 95% of cases of prostate cancer occur, should have an annual prostate examination. This can be performed by a patient's general internist or family practitioner or by a urologist.

To aid in the screening of prostate cancer, a useful test has been developed. This simple blood test is for prostate specific antigen (PSA). The combination of the blood test and the prostate examination provides a useful screen for early disease. Neither test should substitute for the other, and if only one test can be done, it should be the rectal prostate examination. In men with a strong family history of prostate cancer or a long history of benign prostate disease, screening should begin before the age of 50 years. Screening is the only meaningful way to reduce the number of deaths from this disease. To encourage and promote screening, the American Cancer Society sponsors a Prostate Cancer Awareness Week. If a suspicious area is found on examination of the prostate, or if the PSA is elevated, a urologist almost always is consulted. The urologist examines the prostate gland to determine whether a lump is palpable. If a lump is felt, biopsy is performed to determine whether it is malignant. If the lump is benign, nothing further need be done. If it is malignant, the decision-making process must begin. The extent of disease must be carefully determined by staging, and based on the degree and amount of cancer present as well as the age and overall health of the patient, recommendations are made.

Prostate cancer has four stages: A to D. Stage A is actually prostate cancer that is not measurable. That means that the urologist feels no tumor, and the radiologic studies of the prostate gland, the ultrasound examination through the rectum (transrectal ultrasound), and the CT scan show no tumor. A biopsy is then done, usually because of an elevated PSA, and cancer is found. Stage B cancer of the prostate is measurable. The tumor, however, is confined to the gland. This type of prostate cancer is most amenable to surgery. Stage C, cancer of the prostate has broken through the gland and involves other structures in the pelvis, especially the periprostatic lymph nodes (peri, around; prostatic, the prostate). This disease is inoperable and incurable. Some oncologists term prostate cancer that has spread (metastasized) to bone stage D.

What to do when prostate cancer is diagnosed is a difficult question. Most oncologists agree that stages A and B prostate cancer are amenable to removal of the prostate gland. However, this is a major procedure involving opening the patient's abdomen and removing the gland and surrounding structures. It often leaves the patient impotent and, rarely, incontinent of urine. These side effects are anything but minor. The cure rate is clearly improved in patients whose cancer is totally removed by surgery, however. The problem is that the surgery is extensive, and many patients are elderly. Therefore, oncologists must weigh the benefit against the morbidity of the surgery. Radiation therapy to the prostate is about 70% as effective as the operation and causes much less morbidity. However, once the cancer has spread outside the prostate gland, chance of cure is minimal. Therefore, most urologists consider it reasonable to offer this surgery, called a **radical prostatectomy,** to attempt to achieve a cure. Patients must be carefully selected and must understand the likelihood of side effects, postoperative complications, and potential benefit. This is especially important because most patients with cancer of the prostate are elderly, and the benefit in life span may be negligible. If the data can be made clear, however, the decision can be made intelligently, and all parties—urologist, patient, and patient's family—will benefit.

The most common operation performed on the prostate gland is transurethral resection of the prostate (TURP), known popularly as the "Roto-rooter job." This operation, performed through a cystoscope that goes through the urethra in the penis, scrapes out the inside of the prostate gland to relieve obstructive symptoms. It is usually done for benign conditions of the prostate gland and has no meaningful role in the cure of prostate cancer. If cancer of the prostate is causing obstructive symptoms, however, this operation may offer relief. TURP is entirely different from the extensive and aggressive surgery performed for cure of prostate cancer, radical prostatectomy, however.

Because the presence of positive lymph nodes around the prostate gland indicate that the cancer is inoperable and incurable, a good question to ask is how the urologist knows this before doing the operation. The answer is not easy. A CT scan of the pelvis often reveals lymph nodes positive for cancer. If such is the case, the operation is not attempted. The CT scan often misses positive lymph nodes, however, and in that case, the urologist, after beginning the procedure, examines the periprostatic lymph nodes for cancer. If these lymph nodes are positive for cancer, the urologist closes the patient and does not perform the extensive surgery. If they are negative, however, the urologist does perform the radical prostatectomy as planned.

Proving that surgery makes any difference in the outcome of this disease is difficult. Therefore, what does one do about elderly men who have stage A (invisible disease) and stage B (small confined measurable tumors) who do not wish to undergo the extensive surgery? In such cases, radiation therapy given to the prostatic bed can control the disease about as well as surgery. This finding has provoked a controversy as to whether one should operate at all. Patients need all the facts before making such a decision.

Prostate cancer that has spread to bone is a painful disease. Prostate cancer stimulates abnormal bone growth by **blastic metastasis.** Metastatic prostate cancer in bone comes from primary cancer of the prostate that has left the gland and spread to the bone. These metastatic foci (sites; plural of focus) can cause fractures, weakness, and severe pain. The pain can be treated with medication. In addition, prostate cancer is unique among men's cancers in its response to hormonal manipulations. Because the prostate gland grows under the influence of **testosterone,** the male hormone, blocking the action of the testosterone often leads to significant regression of the bony disease. This regression results in marked relief of symptoms and often eliminates the need for narcotics. Testosterone is in the family of male hormones called androgens, so this type of treatment is called **androgenic blockade.**

Effective androgenic blockade is achieved in two ways. The first is to remove the source of testosterone by removing both testicles, an operation termed **bilateral orchiectomy.** Removing a man's testicles is a grave event emotionally. Obviously, impotence is complete, and losing the testes often has enormous negative psychologic effects. However, this operation is easy, quick, inexpensive, and often extremely effective. The second way to achieve androgenic blockade is pharmacologically. Two available drugs can completely block all the effects of testosterone in the body. These two drugs, **leuprolide and flutamide,** are expensive and must be taken until the cancer progresses (grows), and one can only be taken by injection. Because these drugs cause total androgenic blockade, they achieve the same effects as orchiectomy. Patients receiving these medications are totally impotent. The testes are still in place, however, and the emotional impact of the injections may be less than that of the surgery. The patient must decide which option to choose.

Once prostate cancer breaks through the hormonal treatment, no treatment works. The most frequent reason for which I am called to treat this illness is management of pain. As an oncologist, I have extensive experience in pain control. In patients with prostate cancer, however, narcotics work less well than in patients with other tumors. The reason is that tumors in the bone cause inflammation, and narcotics do not have anti-inflammatory activity. Therefore, careful combinations of narcotics and anti-inflammatory agents must be used to treat these symptoms.

Recently, a class of drugs called bisphosphonates was released. These drugs stabilize the bone from destruction by inhibiting the cells that break down bone. These cells, **osteoclasts** (osteo, bone; clast, breakdown) are sensitive to this class of drug. The drugs were approved for the treatment of hypercalcemia (elevated calcium in the blood) of malignancy. One of the drugs, however, pamidronate, has the unique ability to inhibit bone pain caused by cancer that has spread to bone. Although, as I am writing this chapter, pamidronate has not been approved for the treatment of malignant bone pain, it works and it probably is used far more frequently for this unofficial indication than it is for hypercalcemia. Hypercalcemia of malignancy is rarely a clinical problem, whereas bone pain from cancer occurs all the time.

Chapter 7

Cancers of the Stomach, Esophagus, and Pancreas

Few advances in treatment and management of these three cancers have been made over the years. All have poor prognoses. All are cancers of the gastrointestinal system, and all are less common than cancer of the colon and rectum. These tumors always arise from the glands of the inner lining of the organ, and they rarely produce symptoms until it is too late.

My goal in this chapter is to create an understanding of the approach to these tumors and to leave you with general concepts about treatment rather than specifics. The reason is that little can be done other than to remove the cancers surgically. The problem is to determine when to perform major surgery and when to do nothing more than palliation, to minimize discomfort.

CANCER OF THE STOMACH

This is one of the few cancers decreasing in frequency in the Western world. Virtually all other cancers of the bowel are increasing in incidence. This decrease has led to a great deal of investigation into the causes of stomach cancer. The most obvious factor to consider is diet, and unquestionably many opinions exist on the relation of food to the etiology of this malignancy. We still have no clear-cut answers.

Stomach cancer is not only increasing in incidence in Japan, it is a common cancer there. One of the biggest differences between Western and Japanese diets is the smoking of food. Further, the Japanese eat a great deal of salt in their sauces, a finding that has led researchers to believe that salt and byproducts of the smoking of food may be potentially causative in this disease. These hypotheses are unsubstantiated, however.

Another circumstantial dietary factor is the consumption of fresh fruits and vegetables. Vegetarians rarely have this disease, and diets low in vegetables and high in meat seem to be slightly more common in patients with cancer of the stomach. Nonetheless, as with smoked food, a conclusion cannot be drawn.

Because stomach cancer is so common in Japan, the Japanese have developed a nationwide screening program for this disease. This program, which is a large-scale search for stomach cancer with an endoscope, detects 40% of patients with stomach cancer in early stages. Of the 40% whose disease is detected early, 90% are surgically cured. Compare that number with the 5% of patients whose stomach cancer is detected early in the United States; most of the others succumb to their disease. Therefore, who should be screened for this cancer? Given that dietary habit has not been shown to relate to this disease definitely, and dietary habit is an extremely vague characteristic from patient to patient, the entire population of the United States would need to be screened if diet were used as a guide. Therefore, physicians look for certain symptoms that may indicate the presence of this disease.

Obviously, if an ulcer is suspected, a radiographic or endoscopic procedure is ordered. If a gastric ulcer is diagnosed, the treating physician must make sure that the ulcer is not cancer. This can be done by treating the ulcer and proving healing on an x-ray study or performing a biopsy of the ulcer through an endoscope. Both these procedures are safe and easy to perform. Unfortunately, once cancer of the stomach has caused an ulcer, it is usually too advanced to be operable.

Another symptom is a new onset of protracted indigestion. This does not mean if you have indigestion, you need to think about stomach cancer. It does mean that if the way in which food is digested changes, or if the response to food or swallowing changes and persists, one of the foregoing diagnostic procedures is indicated. What should not be done is the routine prescription of antiulcer medications for long periods for nonspecific, undiagnosed symptoms. The most frequent class of drugs abused in this fashion are the H_2 blockers. These drugs (trade names Tagamet, Zantac, and Pepsid) are often prescribed for upset stomach without a diagnosis. Because they work so well, they are often prescribed for protracted periods and may mask symptoms that would lead to a diagnosis of a potentially treatable malignant disease.

Stomach cancer usually has no early warning signs. Routine screening is inappropriate, but the index of suspicion should be high if related symptoms persist. However, there is one exception. **Pernicious anemia,** a disorder in which a protein in the stomach necessary for the absorption of vitamin B_{12} is lost because of loss of the lining of stomach, is associated with an increased incidence of cancer of the stomach. This loss of the inner lining of the stomach is called **atrophic gastritis.** Atrophic gastritis is common, and only a tiny portion of the people, usually elderly, with atrophic gastritis have pernicious anemia, but all patients with pernicious anemia have atrophic gastritis. These patients have a much higher incidence of cancer of the stomach than the general population. This finding has led to a controversy whether these individuals should be routinely screened. Because cancer of the stomach occurs in only a few patients with pernicious anemia, the yield on routine screening is low. Early detection of this disease results in cure, however, whereas late detection does not. Therefore, in patients with pernicious anemia, I recommend that a baseline **gastroscopy** (endoscopic examination of the stomach) be performed, followed by annual gastroscopy. I have detected two stomach cancers in 18 years in patients with pernicious anemia. Both patients are alive and well. One of these patients is one of my dearest friends and was one of America's medical education giants. When I was in New York, we used to have dinner regularly. He was diagnosed as having pernicious anemia 40 years earlier. Vitamin B_{12} injections had been given for the same period of time, and he no longer had evidence of pernicious anemia (completely masked by the B_{12} injections). B_{12} injections do not correct atrophic gastritis, however, nor do they replace the protein necessary for the absorption of vitamin B_{12}. Therefore, they do not decrease the propensity for people with pernicious anemia to develop stomach cancer.

We were at an Italian restaurant on the East side of Manhattan. He was having his favorite spaghetti with garlic and oil, not a particularly difficult food to swallow. I noticed a squint on every mouthful, and knowing about his history of pernicious anemia, asked him what was wrong. His response was that it was a little indigestion that would go away soon. My response was that he was having endoscopy the next morning. Needless to say, the stomach cancer was caught early, and now 12 years later, he still is angry with me for his indigestion associated with having no stomach.

Once stomach cancer is diagnosed, every attempt to remove it should be made. If the disease is beyond the surgeon's ability to eradicate it, chemotherapy can offer an improved life span, but no cure. Various different chemotherapeutic agents have been used with no clear best regimen. Our group is experimenting with 5-fluorouracil (5-FU) and an experimental agent, PALA, which makes 5-FU more potent. It is too early to tell how well these drugs will work.

Some groups have reported excellent response rates with combinations of newer agents. The long-term results are unclear, but what is clear is that there are response rates to chemotherapy. Many of the combinations we use are extremely toxic, whereas others are easier to tolerate. The goals, expectations, and previous responses to therapy must be made clear to patients before subjecting them to treatment. Once these have been explained, however, and the patient expresses a desire to undergo chemotherapy to have life extended, treatment is appropriate. Some patients have good responses; other do not. Patients with good responses live longer with much better quality of life.

The most exciting area of investigation in cancer of the stomach is not with advanced inoperable disease, but with disease that has been operated on but has a high likelihood of recurrence, as determined by **staging** of the disease at operation. This staging involves analysis of the cancer and its characteristics based on the extent of involvement of the wall of the stomach and the surrounding lymph nodes. If the characteristics of the cancer suggest that the tumor is likely to recur, one may ask whether chemotherapy right after surgery or even before surgery would decrease the chance of recurrence significantly. Such treatment should be done on carefully controlled clinical trials, with data from many centers scrutinized carefully. If no such trials are available, the patient must be advised precisely about the goals of treatment. This type of treatment is called **adjuvant** (after surgery in the absence of measurable disease) or **neoadjuvant** (before surgery) chemotherapy. It is impossible to determine whether the chemotherapy is working during the course of treatment because the patient has no evident disease to monitor. If this point is made clear, however, and the patient wants to participate in the trial or undergo the therapy, it is completely appropriate. One group from Germany reported a 33% decrease in cancer recurrence among patients who received intensive chemotherapy after surgery. Some of the treated patients died during treatment. This disease is fatal when it recurs, however, so treatment that decreases recurrence is appropriate. The decision must be made by patients after careful explanations of costs, side effects, goals, and expectations. What would you do?

CANCER OF THE ESOPHAGUS

Unlike cancer of the stomach, a cancer that occurs in an organ with a large volume, esophageal cancers have virtually nowhere to go once they become established, and they usually become evident after it is too late to operate on them. Difficulty swallowing (dysphagia) is the commonest presenting manifestation of cancer of the esophagus. Depending on the size and location of the cancer, the dysphagia usually starts with bulky foods such as meat and later extends to softer foods and liquids. As the tumor enlarges, inability to swallow progresses, and food often is aspirated into the lung. Such aspiration can lead to pneumonias, choking, and even suffocation or asphyxiation. Because the esophagus is a narrow organ, the growing tumor has little place to go, and death occurs early, as a result of starvation, suffocation, or aspiration. Treatment of advanced disease rarely provides much relief and may even increase the symptoms of sore throat and difficulty in swallowing.

Fortunately, cancer of the esophagus is rare. It makes up only 4% of all cancers of the gastrointestinal system, so only about 10,000 cases per year are reported in the United States. The disease is much more common in men than in women; fewer than 25% of cases occur in women. It is more common in elderly patients than in younger people, and it occurs in smokers and drinkers more than in nonsmokers and nondrinkers. The combination of smoking and excessive alcohol intake is especially **synergistic** (additive) in causing cancer of the esophagus. This finding suggests that caustic injury to the esophagus on a regular basis predisposes persons to this disease. In fact, a condition called **Barrett's esophagus,** which is caused by chronic **reflux** (backup) of acid from the stomach to the esophagus, carries a high risk of cancer of the esophagus. Up to 10% of people with this problem develop this type of cancer.

The real goal in the management of this illness is to catch it early enough to operate. The problem is that the disease is not usually **resectable** (completely removable), and because of the location of esophageal cancers, surgery often is necessary to make the patient's life bearable. Further, removal of the esophagus is no small chore. A suitable tube must be created to allow swallowing and to keep oral secretion from entering the lung. Therefore, the surgeon must assess the extent of tumor involvement of the wall of the esophagus as well as the size of the primary tumor. This assessment should be made by a thoracic surgeon with the use of both the endoscope and radiographs of the esophagus. Newer surgical techniques have allowed better tolerance of surgery, and death from the operation itself has decreased from more than 30% to less than 5% in the last two decades. Further, with wider use of endoscopy, more of these lesions are detected earlier, and the cure rate has risen from 2 to 3% to around 10 to 15%. Stage of disease, not location within the esophagus, is the only important variable in determining curability.

Chemotherapy and radiation therapy have a relatively high response rate and offer significant opportunity for palliation, although not for survival or cure. Therefore, to pursue a course of treatment is reasonable as long as patient and family understand the side effects and the goals of such treatment, whether chemotherapy alone or combined chemotherapy and radiation therapy.

Dr. Arlene Forestiere, professor of oncology at Johns Hopkins School of Medicine, has designed a program in which patients with early invasive (the tumor has invaded the wall of the esophagus) cancer of the esophagus are subjected to a short but intensive course of combined and concomitant (given together) chemotherapy and radiation therapy before surgery. This neoadjuvant treatment is used to kill potential disease beyond the surgical field before the removal of the esophagus. So far, 40% of patients treated in this fashion have no evidence of cancer at the time of surgery. The ultimate benefit in survival remains to be seen, but for the first time in the history of this disease, a form of treatment has the potential to increase the cure rate. I strongly recommend that my patients participate in this trial if at all possible. If they cannot participate, I offer them the identical therapy at my institution. All physicians who treat cancer of the esophagus are eagerly awaiting the final results of this trial.

After the chemotherapy is given and the patient has healed from the effects of the treatment, a thoracic surgeon removes the esophagus or the portion of the esophagus containing the cancer. A portion of the stomach is pulled up to act as a food pipe, and the patient is then monitored carefully for signs of cancer recurrence. For the first time, I feel some optimism about this illness and I am grateful to Dr. Forestiere.

For patients with esophageal cancer, gentle management of symptoms and careful attention to the side effects must be part of care. One of the most difficult aspects of this management is to prepare patients and their families for the patient's death. Therefore, physicians should look for this illness if patients have the suggestive symptom of difficulty in swallowing or intolerance to foods.

CANCER OF THE PANCREAS

The incidence of cancer of the pancreas is rising, and survival rates are low. The only hope for cure, as with other gastrointestinal cancers, is surgical removal, and this disease rarely becomes apparent at an operable stage.

One of the problems with this disease arises from the location of the pancreas. Sitting adjacent to the liver, pancreatic cancers grow silently. If a patient with this disease is extremely lucky, the tumor will cause symptoms at a stage where a surgeon can operate, but such is rarely the case. Symptoms are weight loss, jaundice (turning yellow because of obstruction of bile flow), and pain. Pain is almost always a late symptom, and so are the other two. Rarely, however, a surgeon may be asked to evaluate a pancreatic mass at a stage where wide removal of the tumor, which usually requires removal of the pancreas and many surrounding structures, is possible. The operation has a high mortality rate, and usually the tumor recurs.

The incidence of pancreatic cancer increases with age. This cancer is the second commonest malignancy of the gastrointestinal system, second only to colon cancer in incidence. Men develop the disease more than women, and it is more common in New York City Jews and in Israel than otherwise. The incidence in Israel may be partly explained by the higher percentage of cigarette smokers, but Jews in New York do not have a higher incidence of smoking than the general population. Moreover, alcohol seems to synergize with cigarettes in increasing the incidence of this disease, but the causative role is unclear. In addition, **chronic pancreatitis,** which is inflammation of the pancreas, does not seem to be associated with an increased incidence of cancer of the pancreas. Several years ago, coffee was suggested as a predisposing factor in pancreatic cancer, but careful epidemiologic studies have failed to support this position.

Therefore, because one cannot identify a population clearly at risk, screening for this disease is difficult. If a patient consults a physician for symptoms suggestive of pancreatic cancer, the doctor must order a CT scan of the abdomen to look for a pancreatic mass. If a mass is present, a surgeon should be called. If the CT scan is negative, however, another useful test can be done by either a surgeon or a specialist in gastroenterology. This test, endoscopic retrograde cholangiopancreatography is an examination of the pancreatic duct (the portion of the pancreas that empties into the small intestine allowing pancreatic digestive juices to do their work) using an endoscope that enables the physician to look directly into the pancreatic duct and then take a radiograph. The combination of these procedures leads to accurate diagnosis 90% of the time. The CT scan also allows the physician to determine whether liver metastases are present at the time of diagnosis. These metastases, an absolute contraindication to curative surgery, are common in this disease. Nonetheless, a patient who has no evidence of distant spread of cancer must be evaluated for surgery. What often happens in this instance is an operation is performed and the surgeon finds that the tumor is not removable.

Patients with inoperable tumors should be informed of the role of palliative surgery in this disease, to provide symptom relief. Palliation should often be done before symptoms begin. Two of the worst symptoms of pancreatic cancer are obstruction to food flow from the stomach, because of the close proximity of the pancreas to the gastric (stomach) outlet, and jaundice, which turns the patient yellow because of blockage of bile flow from the biliary duct from the liver. The pancreas is also close to the biliary ducts, and the tumor compresses the ducts and so blocks the flow. This debilitating problem can be avoided by intelligent surgery at the time of initial diagnosis.

I routinely insist that two operations be performed when the patient's abdomen is opened and the tumor is found to be unresectable. These procedures are usually technically possible. The first procedure, the **gastroduodenal bypass,** allows food to go directly into the small intestine away from the obstruction of the pancreatic cancer. The second procedure, the **choledochoduodenal bypass,** allows bile to go from the liver to the small intestine without being blocked by the tumor. This combination of procedures does not increase the operative morbidity and provides enormous relief of patients' symptoms.

I wrote a protocol to try a novel combination of chemotherapy for cancer of the pancreas. The study was being performed in about 19 centers nationwide. The early results were encouraging, but minimally so. One of my patients agreed to participate in the trial with this new combination of chemotherapeutic drugs. She had already developed metastases in the liver. I asked a general surgeon to perform the palliative gastroduodenal and choledochoduodenal bypasses. The surgery was performed without difficulty, and the patient's postoperative recovery was short. Chemotherapy was started promptly, but the side effects prompted the patient to stop therapy after 1 month of treatment. It is now 7 months later. She continues to be well without significant symptoms. She is able to eat, her weight is stable, and she is not jaundiced. The location of her tumor would have prevented both these situations had palliative surgery not been done. I am truly sorry that chemotherapy could not have helped her, but surgery surely has improved her life and has decreased the morbidity of her disease.

Chemotherapy for cancer of the pancreas does not appear to work. A rare patient achieves a decrease in tumor, but rarely lives longer as a result of the treatment. Patients who achieve a response to treatment probably have fewer side effects from the disease, however.

Unfortunately, oncologists do not have meaningful therapy for this disease once it has become inoperable. That does not mean that we should not treat patients with new regimens in the setting of a cooperative trial to learn about the effects of new drugs or new combinations of drugs. Without such trials, progress will not be made in the management of this disease.

Chapter 8

Cancers of the Kidney and Bladder

Although cancers of the kidney and bladder are two different diseases, they are closely related because of the functions of these organs. Further, they are both urologic tumors and are both uncommon. Both these tumors can be effectively treated with chemotherapy, but like most solid tumors, they are only curable with surgical removal once they have spread from their primary site (metastasized).

CANCER OF THE KIDNEY

This disease is not a common cancer, but it does cause about 10,000 deaths per year. More than 20,000 new cases of cancer of the kidney are reported annually. The commonest cancer of the kidney is that arising from the kidney parenchyma (tissue) cell itself. This cancer is called **renal cell carcinoma** and it is about twice as common in males as in females. The cause of cancer of the kidney, like that of most cancers, is unknown, but the disease is several times more common in smokers than in nonsmokers. The reason is probably that many of the toxic products of cigarettes are excreted in the urine.

Unfortunately, cancer of the kidney is quiet in its early stages. The location of the kidney makes it uncommon for this tumor to hurt, to cause signs of stretching of the kidney capsule, or to cause bleeding. Kidney cancer often causes microscopic blood in the urine, however. Should this occur in the absence of infection, the physician must look for either cancer of the kidney or cancer of the bladder. Because (microscopic blood in the urine) hematuria is not visible during urination, it is usually detected on routine urinalysis.

When kidney cancer is suspected, a computed tomography (CT) scan of the abdomen should be performed. This scan allows the physician to see a mass in the majority of cases. If cancer of the kidney is suspected, a search for metastases to lung, liver, and brain should be done before surgery. Such metastases make the tumor inoperable. Although some physicians formerly believed that removal of the primary cancer had benefit in the treatment of the metastases, there is no conclusive evidence that this is true, and such major surgery can subject a patient with a manageable terminal illness to extreme morbidity and even mortality. If the primary tumor is causing disabling symptoms, however, especially bleeding, removal of the cancer may be beneficial to the patient. Such decisions must be made on an individual basis, with clear depiction of the outcome, benefits, and risks of such surgery.

Some biologic agents have shown promise in treating this disease. One of these, interferon, has been shown to increase response rates and life span when it is used in combination with other chemotherapeutic agents. A newer compound, interleukin, is being studied at the National Cancer Institute in combination with large doses of other drugs. My cooperative group is currently investigating the combination of 5-fluorouracil, which is given continuously, 24 hours per day, through a port in the chest and a pump attached to the belt, and interferon. We hope that this combination will increase the response rate to this otherwise refractory disease. The National Cancer Institute is using high-dose chemotherapy plus interleukin, a biologic agent that modulates the immune system, in patients with metastatic renal cell cancer. Patients in this study must be in good condition, must have healthy lungs, and must be able to tolerate the treatment. Unfortunately, metastatic cancer of the kidney is a rapidly growing tumor, and patients rarely stay well for long. However, a subset of younger patients can enter this trial. It is only through trials such as these that we will make strides in treating patients with diseases such as cancer of the kidney.

CANCER OF THE BLADDER

Unlike cancer of the kidney, this tumor is easy to detect because of the proximity of the bladder to the urethra (the tube by which urine leaves the body). As a result of this anatomic closeness, bleeding in the urine occurs early. As I mentioned in the section on cancer of the kidney, this symptom, blood in the urine or hematuria, should always prompt a search for cancer of the kidney or bladder if it occurs in the absence of a clearly documented urinary infection, which is vastly more common than either of these cancers.

Bladder cancer is by far the commonest cancer of the urinary tract. It is actually more common than testicular cancer and kidney cancer combined. I exclude prostate cancer from cancer of the urinary tract because the prostate gland has nothing to do with urine formation. About 50,000 cases of cancer of the bladder occur per year in the United States. The disease is more common in older men and 10 times more common in smokers than in nonsmokers. Although the reason for the relationship is not clear, tobacco tar can cause bladder tumors in experimental animal models, and this finding suggests that smoking is an important causative agent in cancer of the bladder.

Once cancer of the bladder is suspected, x-ray procedures can be performed, but **cystoscopy** (cysto-, bladder; -oscopy, examination using a scope) is virtually always necessary. Cystoscopy means insertion of a scope into the bladder to look inside. A urologist performs this procedure in men. In women, it can be performed either by urologists or by gynecologists skilled in the procedure.

A urologist who discovers cancer of the bladder must determine, by biopsy, the depth of penetration into the bladder wall of the tumor. Growth of the tumor into the muscle of the bladder is the single most important indicator of prognosis, especially because superficial cancer of the bladder, which is cancer of the bladder confined solely to the inner lining, can be cured with either simple **ablation** (elimination) with a cystoscope or **fulguration** (cauterization) with electricity.

The use of the laser has made such treatment easier. The urologist must then monitor the patient by means of frequent cystoscopies to look for early recurrences of cancer. These recurrences, if also superficial, can be treated in the same way. Many physicians believe that the instillation of chemotherapy or immunotherapy directly into the bladder can decrease cancer recurrences. If the treating urologist wants to embark on such a program, I believe it is appropriate, as long as the procedure has been fully explained to the patient and consent has been obtained. Data support the concept of such treatment. The instillation of these agents is relatively nontoxic, and the procedure can be performed in minutes on an outpatient basis.

Much more difficult is the decision to operate if the tumor is invasive into the bladder wall, if it is a high-grade lesion, or if it is a superficial cancer that cannot be controlled by local measures. The problem with the decision to operate on patients with these types of bladder cancer is that surgery involves removal of the entire bladder, so urine has nowhere to go once it leaves the kidney. Because urine is made constantly, a person without a bladder would leak urine 24 hours a day. This problem requires the performance of a **diverting ureterostomy,** which brings urine into a bag outside the body. A diverting ureterostomy is similar to a colostomy used for operations on the colon that cannot permit the two ends of the colon to be reunited. Because urine is made so much more frequently than stool, having such a device is a considerable inconvenience to patients.

Another alternative to diverting ureterostomy is to connect the **ureter** (the tube through which urine flows from the kidney to the bladder) to the end of the colon. This procedure is not simple. The liquid urine is not easy to control, leaks frequently, and causes many medical problems. In either event, neither procedure is pleasant, and the decision to operate on patients with such bladder cancers must be made with careful and gentle explanation to patient and family.

No established drugs or combinations of drugs work against advanced cancer of the bladder, but the tumor is responsive, and patients who respond do better during the response. Unfortunately, responses to chemotherapy are usually short-lived, and the 2-year survival of patients with metastatic disease (bladder cancer outside of the pelvis) is minimal.

On the other hand, the cure rate of superficial cancer of the bladder is nearly 90%, and nearly 60% if the disease is invasive and is operated on by **cystectomy** (removal of the bladder).

Chapter 9

Cancer of the Skin

This chapter discusses three types of skin cancer, two of which are similar and one of which, malignant melanoma, is totally different. The three cancers have in common a relation to ultraviolet light—the sun. Skin cancers are far more common than all other malignant diseases combined. Because two commoner types of skin cancer, **basal cell carcinoma** and **squamous cell carcinoma,** are almost always curable when managed reasonably, they are often relegated to management by appropriately trained dermatologists rather than by oncologists.

My goal in this chapter is to describe the means by which we recognize and diagnose these cancers, to stress the early and appropriate management of the two less serious skin cancers and to discuss the management of malignant melanoma.

BASAL CELL CARCINOMA

Basal cell cancer of the skin is the commonest cancer in the world. Well over a half-million cases per year are reported in the United States. Compare this disease with cancer of the lung, which is diagnosed about 175,000 times per year. Basal cell skin cancer is easy to treat and rarely spreads (**metastasizes**). If neglected over a long period, however, cancer can spread to other organs and can become fatal. The length of time required for such an event to occur is usually so long, and the local tissue damage so extensive, that the degree of neglect needs to be staggering.

Basal cell carcinoma develops almost exclusively in white, fair-skinned individuals who are exposed to the sun. The cancer used to be much more common in men than in women but with changes in lifestyle and sun exposure, the sex difference in the incidence of this cancer is disappearing. Many dermatologic oncologists believe that depletion of the ozone layer, with its subsequent loss of ultraviolet blockade, has led to an increased incidence of this cancer. Fortunately, this disease has not become more aggressive, and the death rate in the last decade has not increased.

Because this cancer is directly related to the degree of sun exposure, it is rare in children or young adults. The longer and more frequently one is exposed to the sun, the more likely one is to develop basal cell cancer of the skin. The most frequent site of basal cell cancer is the head and neck, and when the tumor spreads (less than 0.01% of the time), the primary tumor is usually found on the head or neck.

If untreated, basal cell cancer can invade the skin and connective tissue. Huge ulcers may develop and, if further neglected, these ulcers may become infected, leaving even more scarring and contraction. As a result, the cosmetic change can lead to severe morbidity if care is not prompt. The early lesion can be recognized by a small ulcer or **nodule** (raised bump) on the skin, usually around the eyelid or ear lobe. The nose is another frequent site. Over time, this lesion begins to ulcerate, causing small dilated (**varicose**) veins around the border of the lesion. These tiny varicosities, called **telangiectases,** are typical of basal cell carcinoma of the skin. Once these lesions are suspected, a dermatologist should be consulted.

Once the tumor is diagnosed, the goal is complete eradication of the lesion. The actual approach depends on the size of the lesion and the degree of tissue destruction. The choices often are numerous, and the patient and physician should discuss these options with particular attention to the need for preservation of normal skin. Surgery, laser treatment, cautery, freezing, radiation, and topical chemotherapy have all been used with variable degrees of success. These lesions must be treated early and by a dermatologist skilled in management of this cancer.

The prognosis of basal cell cancer is excellent. If the cancer spreads, however, chemotherapy, although effective in controlling the disease for short periods, is strictly palliative (for relief of symptoms), and death is certain. Average survivals vary from 1 to 2 years. In my many years of practice, I have seen only one metastatic basal cell cancer that invaded the bones of the neck in an extremely neglectful construction worker. My goal here is to keep such an occurrence from happening again.

SQUAMOUS CELL CANCER OF THE SKIN

Squamous cell cancer of the skin is the second commonest cancer in the United States. It has virtually the same causes as basal cell cancer. These tumors are faster growing than basal cell cancers and they can metastasize in up to 25% of cases. Like basal cell cancers, however, squamous cell cancers metastasize only after significant periods have elapsed, and one rarely sees metastatic disease in a squamous cell cancer that is not nearly half an inch deep in the skin. Therefore, when squamous cell cancer is suspected, the principles of early treatment outlined for basal cell carcinoma apply.

These cancers are not as typical as basal cell carcinomas. Like basal cell cancer, squamous cell carcinomas tend to ulcerate, but they also tend to crust and scale. Moreover, unlike basal cell cancers, squamous cell carcinomas often arise from premalignant lesions called **keratoses,** common chronic skin lesions in people with excessive sun exposure.

Both these cancers can be prevented by appropriate sun-blocking creams. Golfers, surfers, lifeguards, and construction workers, for example, need to be aware of this problem and should take proper precautions. Unfortunately, these creams are expensive and inconvenient, and their use, although increasing, may not be sufficient to prevent malignant disease. Tanning parlors also are believed to play a role in the development of squamous cell cancer of the skin. Proof is not available, but the type of ultraviolet light used in tanning parlors is the type that predisposes people to keratoses and squamous cell cancer of the skin.

Finally, like basal cell carcinoma, squamous cell cancer of the skin is fatal when it becomes metastatic. Chemotherapy is strictly palliative, and 2-year survivors are rare.

These two cancers, basal cell carcinoma and squamous cell cancer of the skin, are preventable. No one should die of these diseases, and destruction of the skin and underlying tissues should be minimal.

MALIGNANT MELANOMA

Unlike basal and squamous cell cancers of the skin, malignant melanoma is an aggressive and often fatal cancer. Fortunately, most melanomas can be caught early and surgically excised. Once this cancer grows deeply, however, (deep in this discussion here is closer to a millimeter than a centimeter), fatality almost always occurs. Melanoma arises from pigmented moles or freckles. The way to suspect melanoma is to notice a changing, growing, or irregular mole. Any such mole should undergo biopsy by a surgeon or skilled dermatologist, as discussed later.

Melanomas are much more common in white than in black people. Among white people, they are more common in fair-skinned people. Melanomas also may cluster in families, and a prior melanoma in a given individual increases the chance of developing another. Although the disease is uncommon, it is increasing in frequency. Of the approximately 25,000 cases per year reported in the United States, 6000 patients will die of metastatic disease. Proper management can decrease this number.

As just mentioned, once a changing mole is observed, it must undergo biopsy. The single most important factor in the prognosis of melanoma is the total thickness of the lesion. Therefore, the biopsy specimen of a suspected melanoma must include the total thickness of the tumor. Surgical excision and total-thickness core punch biopsy are the only acceptable means of diagnosing these tumors. Partial incisions, shave biopsies, and electrical cautery of melanoma are unacceptable practice.

Once the tumor is excised and melanoma is diagnosed, the tumor must be staged. The staging system for melanoma that is most widely accepted is that of the American Joint Committee on Cancer. Tumor categories are determined by the total thickness of the tumor; the more advanced stages are the thicker tumors. This thickness is from top to bottom of the pigmented lesion and not from side to side. The maximum thickness of the melanoma is measured from the uppermost point of the cancer to the deepest portion of its depth of invasion into the skin. Stages are as follows:

Stage IA: less than 0.75 mm in thickness
Stage IB: 0.76 to 1.5 mm in thickness
Stage IIA: 1.5 to 4 mm in thickness
Stage IIB: more than 4 mm in thickness
Stage III: local lymph node involvement
Stage IV: metastatic disease

The first place of spread of melanoma is to the local or regional lymph nodes. Normally, lymph node involvement is an index of incurability. If only one lymph node is positive for cancer, then surgical excision is still potentially curative. Therefore, a careful search for advanced disease is indicated to avoid unnecessary surgery. A chest radiograph is always indicated to look for silent disease in the lungs. If such disease is found, surgical cure is impossible. Routine laboratory tests should be ordered to assess liver and bone function. If the slightest abnormality is present in either of these blood tests, appropriate radiographs or scans should be obtained. Involvement of bone or liver also precludes a surgical cure. Melanoma also can spread to the esophagus or the stomach. If the patient has difficulty in swallowing, an upper gastrointestinal series (upper GI; radiographs of the stomach and esophagus) should be done. If a suggestion of melanoma is present, an endoscopic examination should be done to perform a biopsy of potential metastasis. If metastases are found, surgical cure is impossible to achieve.

If the patient has no evidence of distant spread of disease, however, complete surgical removal with a margin of appropriate width should be performed. A carefully controlled randomized study compared a surgical margin of 1 or 2 cm (0.5 to 1 inch) with a margin of 4 or 5 cm. The more extensive surgery added nothing to survival, risk, local recurrence, or occurrence of distant metastases. This does not apply to extremely large lesions that require wide excisions to include microscopic surrounding lesions called **satellites.** For primary melanoma less than 1 mm in thickness, which is the most common type of melanoma, however, a 1-cm margin is adequate with a primary closure of the wound (suturing the two ends together to leave a linear scar).

An important exception to the foregoing is that wide excision of the lymph nodes is indicated in patients in whom lymph node metastases is suspected at the time of diagnosis. This operation, **radical lymphadenectomy** (radical, wide; lymphaden, lymph node, -ectomy, removal), is associated with some morbidity because the lymph nodes are responsible for draining fluids in the extremities. Therefore, the performance of a radical lymphadenectomy predisposes patients to swelling of the arms and legs called **lymphedema.** This problem is difficult to control and often requires years of appropriate heavy-support stockings to help to drain the fluid from the tissues of the arms and legs. Consequently, these types of operations are only performed on melanomas of the arms and legs. Further, they should only be performed when the risk of lymph node involvement is high and the patient has no evidence of distant metastatic disease. If a physician suspects lymph node involvement from a melanoma of the leg and the patient already has metastatic disease in the lung, surgical cure is impossible, and the patient should not be subjected to the morbidity of extensive surgery.

Lymphadenectomies are most successful in melanomas of the leg that are larger than 0.75 mm and smaller than 1.5 mm in diameter; that is, stage IB. This group of patients has a near 40% decrease in recurrence rate with prophylactic (preventive) lymphadenectomy. That means that 40% of patients who would subsequently develop distant metastatic disease do not, and 40% of the patients who would otherwise die of metastatic malignant melanoma do not.

Once melanoma is metastatic, it is fatal. Therefore, appropriate early management is essential. Chemotherapy has little benefit in this disease, but some potentially promising treatments are under investigation. These treatments are biologic agents such as interferon and interleukin (see chap. 8). They can trigger the body's immune system to attack the melanoma, and with the aid of chemotherapy, these agents have been able to achieve remissions in this otherwise refractory disease. Recent evidence suggests that **adjuvant chemotherapy** at the time of surgery (adjuvant meaning to prevent potential disease) in the absence of distant metastases may improve the management of malignant melanoma. No evidence indicates that chemotherapy for malignant melanoma has any benefit in survival or quality of life. Therefore, I only treat patients with metastatic malignant melanoma with participation in a cooperative group trial of investigational agents or investigational combinations of older agents.

Advanced melanoma can spread virtually anywhere in the body. When it has spread to local lymph nodes, with the exception of stage IB melanomas of the leg, it causes distant metastases 90% of the time. Therefore, a pigmented lesion that is irregular, changing, or growing should be evaluated. After evaluation, if melanoma is suspected, it should undergo full-thickness biopsy. When biopsied it must be a full-thickness biopsy with any other procedure totally unacceptable. If melanoma is diagnosed, it should be removed by a surgeon skilled in current techniques of melanoma surgery.

Chapter 10

Ovarian Cancer

Ovarian cancer is extremely sensitive to chemotherapy, and many advances have been made in its treatment. Further, during the last 10 years, we have learned that this cancer has a huge familial pattern, and high-risk groups have been defined.

Cancer of the ovary is the sixth most common cancer in women. However, it is the fourth most common cause of death from cancer in women and the commonest cause of death from gynecologic cancer. Ovarian cancer increases in frequency with advancing age, and in women over 60 years old, it is the commonest gynecologic cancer. More than 20,000 new cases per year are diagnosed in the United States. More than 60% of these patients die of ovarian cancer. Because these numbers are significant, a program to detect early cancer of the ovary is badly needed. Even today, no good program for early detection of ovarian cancer exists.

For more than 20 years, a registry existed for familial ovarian cancer, but it did not receive much use. In the late 1980s however, comedienne Gilda Radner died of ovarian cancer. Her candid discussion of her illness, along with the generous support of her husband, Gene Wilder, prompted articles in major newspapers around the United States, and many families in whom ovarian cancer is clustered were identified. As a result, it was learned that the highest risk factor for cancer of the ovary is either a history of ovarian cancer or a mother or sister with the disease. Nonetheless, in families in whom several direct blood relatives, such as aunts, grandmothers, and cousins, have had the disease, the risk is clearly elevated. Further, in the breast/ovarian cancer syndrome, the two cancers cluster in a given family.

SCREENING

Unfortunately, no single good screening tool is available to determine whether a woman has cancer of the ovary in the absence of any symptoms. The blood test for CA 125, which is a biologic marker for cancer of the ovary, is an excellent tool for monitoring the progress of treatment. Unfortunately, it is too nonspecific for use as a large-scale screen. What this means is that too many other causes of elevated CA 125 beside ovarian cancer are possible to make the test specific, and too many patients with ovarian cancer have a normal CA 125 to make the test sensitive.

Another useful tool is pelvic ultrasound examination. This completely safe and noninvasive procedure, available in most radiology departments, is sensitive to ovarian masses. The problem is that many ovarian masses are completely benign, and the pelvic ultrasound examination, if used as a screening tool, would detect minor abnormalities such as benign cysts. A physician who is screening a patient for cancer of the ovary and who notes **positive** signs must prove that the patient does not have cancer. Therefore, countless, albeit minor, operations, would be performed if the pelvic ultrasound examination were used as a screen.

The same principle applies to the physical examination performed by a gynecologist. Positive findings on pelvic examination are evaluated by ultrasound. If the index of suspicion is high, the ovary may have to be examined either by exploratory surgery or by the use of **laparoscope,** a device that permits clear visualization of the pelvic organs. Although this surgical procedure is minor, it still involves risks of organ injury and anesthesia. Any surgery should be avoided if possible, and physicians do not want to investigate benign disease surgically more often than necessary. Ovarian cancer can be fatal, however. Therefore, women at high risk should have an annual pelvic examination and either a CA 125 determination or a pelvic ultrasound examination, or both. If an index of suspicion exists, a diagnosis of ovarian cancer should be excluded. If **any** of the screens are positive, the ovary must be carefully examined to make sure that no tumor is present. If a woman falls into the category of a familial ovarian cancer syndrome, and she is the sister or daughter of two or more first-degree relatives with the disease, her ovaries should be removed prophylactically (as a preventive measure) because she will have about a 50% chance of developing ovarian cancer and more than a 60% chance of dying of the disease.

ROLE OF THE OVARIES AFTER REPRODUCTION

Although the ovaries are not essential organs for life, they produce the female hormone, **estrogen.** Data on the protective effects of estrogen on heart disease, by delaying hardening of the arteries, and on osteoporosis have led gynecologists increasingly to prescribe estrogen replacement to postmenopausal women. Eliminating the major source of estrogen from premenopausal women by removing their ovaries therefore has a negative effect on the health of these women. Gynecologists believe that the risk of ovarian cancer is far less than the risk of serious heart disease or disabling osteoporosis resulting from estrogen deprivation. Therefore, when a woman has a hysterectomy for reasons completely unrelated to her ovaries, the ovaries are often left behind to provide estrogen, even though the possibility of conception is eliminated by removal of the uterus and the fallopian tubes. To the oncologists, this situation is confusing because ovarian cancer is often fatal, and preventing ovarian cancer is a prime consideration from our vantage point. Therefore, decisions about removing the ovaries must be made on an individual basis.

At present, I do not recommend that premenopausal women who must undergo hysterectomy have their ovaries removed as well. I believe, however, that the risk of ovarian cancer in postmenopausal women is high enough that, if a hysterectomy is going to be performed, the ovaries should be removed at the same time. Further, in postmenopausal women, estrogens can easily be replaced by oral medication. Because the same applies to premenopausal women, it then becomes the patient's decision, along with that of her gynecologist, whether the ovaries should be left in place or removed with the uterus. No consensus exists.

DIAGNOSIS AND STAGING

Whenever a patient has an ovarian mass, the diagnosis of cancer must be excluded. This is true whether the mass is discovered by physical examination, radiograph, or ultrasound. A gynecologist investigates the mass, usually either by laparoscopy, in which a tube allows the surgeon to enter the pelvis, to look at the ovary, to obtain a specimen for biopsy from a suspicious area or mass, or by opening the patient's abdomen and examining the ovary (or ovaries) directly. If an open operation is performed, the gynecologist usually suspects that a tumor is present. This does not mean that a malignant tumor, which only can be determined after biopsy, is present, but one must be prepared for such an event.

If the tumor is found to be malignant, the gynecologist should be prepared to perform a complete staging procedure, including removal of both ovaries, the uterus, and the fallopian tubes. In addition, the lymph nodes around the aorta that drain the pelvis and the connective tissue of the intestines, called the **omentum,** also should be removed. This last procedure is called an **omentectomy** (omentum, connective tissue of bowel; -ectomy, removal). Finally, if the intestines are involved, a partial bowel resection may be performed. This complicated operation requires special skill. In such cases, a gynecologic oncologist, who is trained in treating malignant diseases of the female organs, must be ready to assist in the operation. If such an individual is not available, a gynecologist able to perform the operation must be available, or the patient should be transferred to an institution where the appropriate procedure can be performed. The wrong operation can hinder the patient's chances of cure and may interfere with a second operation.

TREATMENT

The best way to cure ovarian cancer is to remove it surgically. Unfortunately, such is not the case in the majority of ovarian cancers, and medical oncologic therapy must be part of the treatment plan.

Ovarian cancer completely confined to the ovary is called stage I ovarian cancer. Unlike with other tumors, however, several types of stage I cancer are recognized. The reason is that ovarian cancer can produce fluid that contains cancer cells. These cancer cells, when spread around the pelvis or abdominal cavity, can grow as new foci (sites) of cancer and therefore require additional therapy when present. To clarify stage I ovarian cancer, it must be divided into three substages. Ovarian cancer completely confined to the ovary, with no fluid or tumor through the capsule (external border of the ovary) is stage IA cancer of the ovary. Surgical removal of this type of cancer virtually always cures the disease. Unfortunately, this stage is rare. Stage IB ovarian cancer is the same as stage IA, but both ovaries are involved. The management of stage IB disease is the same as that of stage IA, and it has almost the same prognosis. Beyond stage IB disease, the management of ovarian cancer becomes more complex.

Ovarian cancer that has invaded the capsule of the ovary or that has spilled fluid with cancer cells into the abdomen is called stage IC disease. This stage implies that the visible tumor itself is totally confined to the ovary, but because of the potential for these microscopic cells in the fluid to take hold and to grow, additional therapy usually is recommended. Generally, this additional therapy is **adjuvant chemotherapy,** which is the treatment of potential disease. In patients with ovarian cancer, adjuvant chemotherapy has the potential to prevent the recurrence of disease. If cancer recurrences are prevented by adjuvant chemotherapy, the treatment has effectively cured a patient who would otherwise have had a relapse.

Ovarian cancer is sensitive to chemotherapy, and with newer agents that have even greater activity against the disease, the outlook is improving all the time. The problem with such therapy is that it is extremely toxic. The decision-making process is difficult when treating women who are likely to be cured with surgery alone. Therefore, oncologists must clarify the patient's options. Room for dogma exists when the use of treatment is clearly beneficial. In many stages of the disease, however, the use of treatment has either a marginal effect or an insignificant benefit. Failure to clarify these findings to the patient abdicates a physician's responsibility in the management of this disease. In general, a woman with ovarian cancer wants to do whatever is necessary for cure. What we need to bring into perspective is avoiding toxic treatments that cannot offer an improved outcome.

Stage II disease is the rarest of all stages. This consists of tumor in one or both ovaries that has extended into the pelvic structures. The reason that this is so rare is that when ovarian cancer extends beyond the ovary, it usually begins to involve structures outside the pelvis as well. This involvement occurs early. Once ovarian cancer is outside the pelvis, it is either stage III or stage IV disease. Stage III ovarian cancer is tumor involving the abdomen, and stage IV ovarian cancer is tumor involving distant organs such as the liver or lung. Stage IV disease has a worse prognosis than stage III disease. Sometimes, stage III ovarian cancer, which has spread beyond the ovary to involve the abdomen, becomes extensive. When this happens, a large amount of fluid is often produced. If the fluid is extensive enough to cause swelling of the abdomen, the patient can have fluid around the lung as well. This fluid, called a **pleural effusion,** (the pleura is the lining of the lung), may or may not contain malignant cells. If the fluid does contain malignant cells, the stage goes from stage III to IV, but if the fluid in the lung does not contain malignant cells, it is called a sympathetic effusion and remains stage III disease. Although the treatment is not much different for the two stages, the prognosis is worse if the disease involves liver or lung (stage IV).

These advanced stages of ovarian cancer require the cooperation of both surgeons and oncologists. In some institutions, gynecologic oncologists perform the surgery and administer the chemotherapy. In other places, medical oncologists administer the chemotherapy after the surgery is performed. Both modalities of treatment, surgery and chemotherapy, are necessary to treat patients with advanced ovarian cancer.

In ovarian cancer, the approach to surgery is extremely important. The reason is that the less cancer left behind, the more likely the patient will do well with **medical** treatment. Although this idea seems logical, it is not the case with most tumors. Therefore, the role of the surgeon in patients with cancer of the ovary, especially patients with stage III disease, is to remove as much tumor as possible, a process called **debulking.**

Because the spread of this disease through the abdomen often leaves thousands of tiny tumor implants on the bowel and the connecting structures of the intestines, the skill required to perform this maximal debulking is specialized. In fact, in advanced stages of ovarian cancer, removing every last bit of tumor is usually not possible. Therefore, a gynecologic oncologist should be available to assist with the surgery. Special, usually electrical, tools to eradicate tiny implants require special skill and a superior knowledge of abdominal anatomy.

Once the surgery is performed, and a patient with ovarian cancer is referred to the medical oncologist, the medical oncologist asks whether maximal debulking has been accomplished. If the surgeon says that visible disease was eradicated, then the medical oncologist knows that cure is possible. This, of course, refers to stage III disease in which the tumor is confined to the abdomen. Metastatic disease is not operable. Therefore, in a woman with stage III ovarian cancer who has undergone maximal tumor debulking, intensive postoperative treatment should be administered. In fact, the most intensive chemotherapy tolerable should be given. About 25% of patients with stage III cancer of the ovary are curable (when maximal debulking is possible), and only 3 to 5% of patients with stage IV disease are curable (maximal debulking is not possible).

The chemotherapy for cancer of the ovary has changed drastically in recent years. When I was in medical school, the major agent was an oral drug with limited activity. Responses were routine, but cures in patients with any degree of disease left behind after surgery were rare. Patients were operated on by their gynecologists, and adjuvant chemotherapy was left to clinical investigators, who were then trying to improve the outcome of patients whose cancer had spread past the ovary at the time of surgery.

In the late 1970s, the platinum compounds became available. These agents displayed activity against a variety of tumors, especially germ (reproductive) cell tumors. These tumors, which arise from organs of the reproductive system, are all sensitive to chemotherapy.

The first platinum compound to be commercially available was cisplatin. This drug, which is highly active against many cancers, was extremely toxic when it was first released. The reason for the marked toxicity was the limited knowledge of how to protect patients against nausea, vomiting, and kidney disease. Platinum is a heavy metal and is toxic to the kidney. It is also extremely nauseating. Oncologists soon learned that giving the platinum agent with a large volume of fluid limited the toxicity of the drug. Nonetheless, severe nausea was a major problem. Then several years ago, a drug in a new class of antinausea medication was released. This drug, ondansetron (Zofran), is remarkable for its ability to block the brain's perception of nausea without causing drowsiness. The drug is nontoxic, well tolerated by most patients, and usually completely effective. It has completely changed oncologists' ability to deliver higher doses of chemotherapy to patients with platinum-sensitive tumors.

After development of platinum agents, studies began to use different doses of these drugs combined with other agents. For the first time, cures were seen in patients with stage III and IV ovarian cancer. Cure is rare in stage IV disease that has spread outside the abdomen, and although uncommon in stage III disease (only 25%), it is certainly better than no cure at all. Stage III disease is ovarian cancer that has spread to the abdominal cavity. This includes the small and large bowel, stomach, surface of the liver, and walls of the abdomen. Implants of cancer are seen by the operating gynecologist at surgery. If proper surgery is done, as many of these implants as possible are removed during the surgery, and then the patient is allowed to heal. Studies have shown that the best combination of chemotherapeutic drugs to give at this time (immediately after healing from surgery) consists of a platinum agent and cyclophosphamide. When these drugs are given together, an oncologist can monitor the patient with computed tomography (CT) scans of the abdomen and blood tests using the marker CA 125. If the CA 125 falls rapidly after the administration of chemotherapy, prognosis begins to improve. Further, if CA 125 falls to a normal level, it can be used at a later time as a marker of cancer recurrence should the level rise again.

The patient typically receives six cycles of treatment. Treatment is given intravenously and usually requires hospitalization because of the large volumes of fluid required to protect against the kidney toxicity of cisplatin. Moreover, constant antinausea medication is required. Because cisplatin also is toxic to the nerves, the dose of cisplatin is the limiting factor on how much chemotherapy the patient can receive. A few years ago, a related drug, called an **analog,** of cisplatin was developed called carboplatin. This drug is much less toxic to the kidney and much less nauseating, but it is more toxic to the bone marrow. Oncologists can protect patients against bone marrow toxicity, however. Excellent antibiotics protect against infections when the white blood cell count is extremely low, and injections can stimulate the bone marrow to make white blood cells after chemotherapy has halted white cell production. When the platelet count is low, platelets can be transfused. Therefore, doses can be escalated as tolerated by the patient. I have been able to administer twice the equivalent dose of carboplatin to patients as cisplatin. I have thereby increased the number of patients who have sustained complete remission. The data still need to be reviewed, to determine the effect of this type of dose escalation.

If oncologists normally use a dose "X" for a given disease, "1.5X or 2X" is often better. In ovarian cancer, such is the case. Therefore, if I were able to use "X" amount of cisplatin and wanted to use "2X", I could not because of the toxicity. Such is not the case with carboplatin. It is possible, and even safe, with careful monitoring to use "2X" and even "3X or 4X" amount of carboplatin. Therefore, in women able to tolerate dose escalation, I used a fixed dose of cyclophosphamide plus a high dose of carboplatin. The treatment is given every 3 weeks for six cycles (one treatment is a cycle). The patient's blood is monitored at least weekly, and when the carboplatin dose is escalated, I often check the patient's blood three times per week. Prophylactic antibiotics and blood products are given as needed. Most patients tolerate the therapy well.

At the end of the chemotherapy, the CT scans of the abdomen and pelvis are repeated, and CA 125 is monitored again. If the patient has no evidence of disease, the patient is said to be in complete clinical remission. However, there still may be evidence of microscopic disease in the abdomen, and it would cause a relapse in the future. In patients with ovarian cancer, therefore, oncologists often recommend a procedure known as a **second-look operation.** Such an operation is done after the completion of chemotherapy for disease known to be present. When a second-look operation is done, oncologists do not know whether any disease is present. All the staging after the chemotherapy, including the CA 125 determination, is completely negative for cancer. What oncologists are doing is determining whether microscopic or minimal residual disease is present at this point.

Second-look procedures for ovarian cancer have been a subject of debate for at least three decades. Proponents of the procedure probably outnumber those who believe that the operation's usefulness is limited. To reiterate, the following must be present for a patient with ovarian cancer to be considered for second-look surgery:

1. On physical examination, including gynecologic examination of the pelvis, the patient must have absolutely no evidence of disease.

2. All elevated tumor markers must have returned to normal. (In this case, it is usually just CA 125.)

3. All nonsurgical tests such as CT scans or magnetic resonance imaging must show no evidence of disease.

The surgical procedure performed for a second look should, in most cases, be done by the surgeon who performed the original surgery for the primary ovarian cancer. The reason is that, in the healing process of a major operation, anatomic changes occur. The operating surgeon who performed the first operation is better able to see, in a second operation, whether significant changes have occurred.

With the advent of endoscopic operative procedures in the abdomen, (remember the endoscope is like a telescope that allows the surgeon to see the pelvic organs close up) the actual surgery can be performed with tools that fit through the endoscope. Actual major surgery can thereby be avoided, and a second-look operation can now be performed with an incision small enough to admit only the endoscope. With this tool, unless significant scarring (usually referred to as **adhesions**), is present from the original surgery, the surgeon is able to sample any suspicious areas for biopsy, take samples of any fluid in the abdomen and look for malignant cells, actually add solution to the abdomen and suck it back through the endoscope to determine whether the fluid picks up any malignant cells, and take biopsy specimens of any suspicious areas around the bowel and its connecting tissues. Moreover, if the surgeon sees any lymph nodes that drain the abdomen or pelvis, those nodes can be sampled for biopsy or removed.

After the operation, all specimens are sent to the pathology department to look for evidence of recurrent cancer. Two possibilities exist: the specimens can all be negative for tumor; or evidence of residual cancer can be present. If the operation is completely negative for cancer, the woman's prognosis becomes much better. Even more importantly, however, if the pathologist's report shows washings positive for cancer or evidence of minimal residual disease after the surgery, some women can be cured by additional chemotherapy at that time. Rarely does significant harm come from the surgery, and there sometimes is significant benefit. As a patient, which would you choose?

A promising chemotherapeutic agent, paclitaxel (Taxol), comes from the bark of the Pacific yew tree and has excellent ability to block the growth of cancer cells. This drug is toxic and needs to be monitored carefully. Because of its intense activity against ovarian cancer, however, it is currently being studied in combination with the platinum compounds, which to date have been the most active drugs against this tumor, as initial therapy for this disease. Taxol already has been shown effective in some cases of recurrent ovarian cancer, it has replaced cyclophosphamide as the agent of choice in combination with platinum agents for women with ovarian cancer as initial therapy. Taxol represents an exciting addition to our armamentarium against this disease. I have treated three women with this combination, and all are alive, well, and free of disease. We already know that women who have a minimal amount of disease present, as noted at a second-look operation, can be cured with additional chemotherapy. If we have a new drug that is different from the drugs she already has received, this new drug may be even more effective at offering a cure than the drugs used previously.

It will take time to see what role Taxol will play. Meanwhile, the approach to treatment of a woman with this ovarian cancer needs to be aggressive. One of the most gratifying events for me as an oncologist is to tell a woman, 2 to 3 years from her last course of chemotherapy, that she is probably cured.

To conclude, cancer of the ovary will likely become one of the most curable solid tumors in medical oncology. As our techniques for removing disease at surgery continue to improve along with the advent of more active agents, the approach to this illness in an attempt to offer cure will become more successful. In the meantime, we need to improve our ability to detect the tumor earlier and find better ways to screen high risk women. Nonetheless, the outlook for treatment is becoming more and more optimistic, and I believe this disease will not be the killer it is today by the turn of the century.

Chapter 11

The End of Life: Terminal Disease

Terminal disease is a difficult topic that is painful for most people. It is impossible to discuss with parents, regardless of how old the child is. Nonetheless, it is one of the most important aspects of an oncologist's job because, in many cases in clinical oncology, the situation becomes hopeless, and meaningful life in any fashion no longer is possible. In such circumstances, our primary goal becomes control of pain and maintenance of comfort. Preparation of the patient and family for the imminent event—death—accompanies this goal.

STORY OF TWO PATIENTS

I recently lost two patients, both of whom I had taken care of for a long time. In one case, the situation was hopeless from the beginning. The other case was a treatment failure and a great disappointment to all of us caring for him. I would like to relate their stories to you to help you to understand what I believe are the options for a patient who is going to die no matter what further treatments are given. The issue of death has only recently become a major area of discussion in medicine in the United States.

Until recently, not doing things to keep patients alive was anathema. Concerns about narcotic addiction were actually part of care plans for the terminally ill. Thankfully, such is no longer the case.

The first of these two patients was a 29-year-old woman with metastatic breast cancer. She had been operated on 1 year before coming to see me. After her surgery, she received adjuvant chemotherapy because of several positive lymph nodes. Up to that point, her medical care had been delivered at another institution, and it had been impeccable. When the patient arrived in my office, metastatic disease already had been diagnosed by her family doctor. The cancer had spread to her bone marrow.

Metastatic breast cancer, no matter where the metastases are, is fatal. We had to start our relationship with that fact. One does not need to dwell on the hopeless, however, when an illness is still treatable. To that end, after the extent of her disease was determined, I offered to treat her with chemotherapy as part of a protocol through the Middle Atlantic Oncology Program, the cooperative group in which I participate. When we started therapy, the patient was told clearly that there was virtually no chance of cure. However, I told her that response rates were high. If she responded, it was likely that her life could be prolonged considerably. At the same time, the quality of her life would be much better. She never heard me.

As the months went on, more and more of the disease disappeared. By the end of a year of therapy, the patient had no evidence of disease. All her pain had disappeared. Her bone marrow had become normal, with no evidence of cancer. She was in complete remission, with a 100% chance of relapsing somewhere in the not too distant future. This fact was carefully explained. The difference between remission and cure was explained over and over. She never heard.

Finally, more than 18 months after I met her, the patient began having headaches. These were new headaches, and I knew what they meant—the cancer had spread to the brain. Radiation therapy to the brain can be given to help shrink the tumor and to alleviate some of the discomfort. However, there is no chance for meaningful survival. Continuous morphine was given by a catheter (Portocath) that allows access to the veins so patients do not have to be stuck over and over again. This device can be used for the administration of intravenous medications, for drawing blood, and for administering transfusions, and it makes the lives of both patient and physician easier. A tranquilizer and sleep inducer were given for anxiety and sleep. Then, as we instituted all our measures for comfort, her parents arrived. In 18 years of doing this job, I have not learned how to prepare parents for the death of a child. I know how impossible it would be for me. Yet, it is clearly part of the job and an important part. Unrealistic attempts at treatment can turn a sad and terminal case into a horror story.

The patient's mother wanted a second opinion, even though the brain scan showed more than 40 sites of metastatic breast cancer. The mother would not allow us to order "no CPR"—a common order that tells the doctors and nurses **not** to resuscitate a patient who stops breathing or whose heart stops. This well-meaning lady who genuinely loved her daughter actually wanted us to put the young woman on a respirator. I refused to accept her wish. CPR in patients with metastatic cancer has no hope of success, if survival past hospitalization is taken as an end point. This patient, whose death was imminent, could not have survived the respirator. Coaxing on the part of her husband and other children was necessary to make this woman see how horrible it would be for her daughter. The mother's sadness was immeasurable, and the patient finally died, pain free, in her sleep, 4 days after admission to the hospital.

Before I tell you about the second patient, I want to discuss the continuous use of narcotics through an indwelling intravenous line like the Portocath. Not all terminally ill patients who are in pain have to be in the hospital. In either the home or hospital setting, this marvelous device can allow the patient and caregiver to administer enough narcotic to maintain a pain-free state. This concept, patient-controlled analgesia, allows the individual to control pain at the end of life. It avoids the practice of painful intramuscular injections of narcotics to control pain, the standard of care until recently. How stupid it is to order painful injections for a terminally ill patient and make them wait for the next injection. Thankfully, this practice is now rare. Pain control means pain control. It supersedes all other goals in this setting, and the best way to be sure that you have handled the situation adequately is to ask the patient.

The second patient illustrates a situation opposite to that of the first patient, that of a completely treatable disease, albeit one with a guarded prognosis. This patient was a splendid sixty-one-year-old-man with acute myelogenous leukemia. This disease is curable. Although only a minority of patients are cured, the majority go into a complete remission, and during that remission are well and can live normal lives.

John, as I refer to him, came to me more than 2 years before his death. The diagnosis of acute leukemia was absolutely unquestioned. At that time, we were participating in a cooperative group study with Adria laboratories, to examine the efficacy and toxicity of a new drug for acute leukemia. John was selected to receive the new drug. The initial therapy was remarkably easy. He sailed through his initial month in the hospital and had only limited toxicity. A beautiful complete remission ensued. Following the complete remission, another course of chemotherapy was given to consolidate our initial success. Again, he sailed through his treatment. He did so well with the initial course of treatment that the second treatment, the consolidating treatment, was given at home. I even remember his calling me to ask whether it was OK to have sexual intercourse during the chemotherapy. Of course, I answered that it was fine. Shortly after the start of the consolidating therapy, John was admitted with sepsis, which is a severe systemic infection caused by blood-borne bacteria. Once again, he responded beautifully to antibiotics. Again, a complete remission occurred, and he was discharged to home. The initial second remission follow-up was heralded by a complete lack of complications. Our visits became less frequent. John decided to start traveling. On a trip to the Eastern shore of Maryland, while diving for crabs, he ruptured an eardrum. An ear, nose, and throat specialist solved the problem. We agreed that diving was no longer permissible.

John's care became routine. Then one day, he was found unconscious at home. Unknown to all of us, he had suffered a subdural hematoma, which is a collection of blood beneath the surface of the lining of the brain, during the diving accident. This hematoma gradually increased the pressure in his head until he suddenly became unconscious. Once again, with the help of a neurosurgeon, John recovered completely and his life returned to normal. He and his wife decided that he should claim disability and quit his job. He had no limitations in activity and took numerous trips. He insisted on handling the majority of the household chores.

Then, on a routine visit to my office, leukemic cells began to appear on the glass slide that I used to examine John's blood. Clearly, this represented seriously bad news, because the relapse of acute leukemia is rarely curable. In our initial encounter, I had already explained that a relapse of this disease meant that death was nearly certain.

Our next visit was late in the summer. John had been working in his rose garden and had been stuck by a thorn. Because leukemia interferes with the production of normal white blood cells (see Chap. 5), normal immune responses to infection do not occur. Where the rose thorn had punctured his skin was severely inflamed. Yet John was well and wanted to get on with his daily activities. His mood never changed from positive and optimistic. On seeing the wound on his leg, I admitted John to the hospital, cultured the wound, had a biopsy performed. The infection was caused by a fungus called aspergillus, which does not usually cause disease in people with normal immune systems. In John, however, with this relapse of leukemia, if the fungal infection went untreated, a severe, eventually fatal infection would occur. Intensive treatment with a potent and toxic antifungal agent was given in the hospital. Topical therapy to the skin was administered, and slowly but surely the injured area began to heal. The leukemia continued to worsen, and the issue of what to do with now relapsed leukemia had to be faced.

John was a fighter, and he asked what was maximally available for someone in "his boat." I called several of my friends in the field of leukemia treatment research. Fortunately, one of the world's authorities on leukemia therapy is in Baltimore. Together, we went over John's case and designed an intensive regimen that we believed would offer him the possibility of a reasonable remission. Don't ask what a reasonable remission means in this disease, because little evidence indicates that long-term survival is possible. If untreated, however, relapsed leukemia kills in weeks. John opted to start treatment, but he wanted to take a trip to Arizona with his wife. They had a wonderful time. We kept in close contact during the 10 days of his trip.

John was admitted to the hospital from the airport on his return. The treatment was extremely toxic, but as before, this wonderful and vigorous fighter weathered the storm well. However, the fungus that had infected his skin earlier had moved to his lung, and we had to fight to keep his breathing stable. As we reached 42 days after the completion of the chemotherapy and waited for the normal bone marrow to return, John's breathing became unacceptably shallow, and an emergency decision had to be made. Should we do nothing and let him die in minutes, or should we put him on a respirator to assist his breathing and hope that the next few days would herald the return of normal bone marrow and that his immunity would destroy the fungus and that his breathing would become acceptable?

John, his family, and I had agreed that, should a respirator become necessary, we would allow him to die peacefully. Yet, I could not stand allowing him to die with this thread of hope that a return of normal bone marrow function might allow his recovery. I asked the family to let me put him on a respirator. They agreed. During the next 2 days, a desperate attempt was made to keep John alive. Finally, the respirator and our heroic efforts failed, and this beautiful, strong, courageous man died. The last blood count, done on the day of his death, showed a resurgence of leukemic cells. It would not even have mattered.

Why do I present these two cases? Because, in my opinion, they represent the extremes of what to do in the case of terminal disease. Both patients died with their families experiencing intense anxiety. The young lady with breast cancer never came to grips with the inevitability of her death, and the wonderful man with leukemia died a virtually hopeless death on a respirator. What can and should be done as death becomes inevitable?

The first thing that patients and physicians must gain in this setting is understanding and agreement that meaningful survival no longer is possible. The argument that "one never knows" is simply not viable because we usually know that it will not be possible to provide any more meaningful treatment. An understanding among family, patient, and physician can then be reached.

CARE OF THE TERMINALLY ILL

At this juncture, it is reasonable to spell out the options for creating a comfortable and dignified end. Palliation of symptoms should be made clear to the patient. Palliation means to provide relief. In the setting of terminal and hopeless disease, it should take precedence over all other concerns. Addiction is of no concern. Pain medicine should keep pain from occurring, not take away pain after it becomes intense. There is simply no reason for patients in this state to suffer, nor is there justification for requiring a waiting period for relief of pain. Nurses or patients themselves can be allowed to titrate (adjust up or down) the dose of narcotics to control pain.

If severe pain is present, two major types of drugs should be used. First, long-acting oral narcotics provide mobility and freedom from discomfort. These drugs have a life in the blood of more than 8 hours, so merely taking them twice or three times daily provides adequate pain relief to allow a productive and enjoyable life. These drugs also can be easily titrated upward as shorter-acting narcotics become more necessary to alleviate pain that occurs throughout the day.

Inevitably, however, as cancer progresses, oral agents no longer control pain. Once again, use of the Portocath, the permanently implanted intravenous access device, becomes useful. When such a device is in place, continuous or intermittent morphine can be delivered into the bloodstream by a pump worn on the patient's belt or strap. This provides effective pain relief during the end stages of terminal cancer. Weeks of comfort at home can be achieved. Using a demand button on the pump, the patient can add drug in small quantities to provide necessary comfort. Some of my patients over the years actually enjoyed vacations with their families while using such devices. This principle is called patient-controlled analgesia. More than 95% of patients can maintain functional lifestyles using this method of pain control. Further, for patients who do not have a permanent catheter, the medication can be delivered intravenously by pump. We have made a great stride forward in the management of pain, especially chronic pain, in patients whose disease is not going to go away.

Physicians and patients must remember that when chronic or continuous pain relief is necessary and narcotics are used on a routine basis, constipation occurs. The constipation caused by long-term narcotic use can be debilitating. Preventing this problem is a lot easier than treating it. One of the most useful tools is a glass of prune juice in the morning. It's not a prescription drug, but is remarkably useful and best of all cheap. The important thing to remember is to remember to take it. The relief this provides to the terminally ill patient is immeasurable. A high-fiber diet also is useful. A patient's appetite may be poor, however, and adherence to a prescribed diet may not be possible. To that end, the use of a bowel regulator or stool softener is very useful. An agent that I prescribe routinely is a liquid called lactulose. This compound, a large sugar, draws water into the colon and makes the stool softer as it regulates the movement of the bowel.

Dying patients are not dead. Their care requires specialized interaction. Earlier this year, I listened to a medical grand rounds at Franklin Square Hospital Center given by a nurse thanatologist. This woman taught me some important insights into the care of the dying patient. Simple, almost obvious lessons were learned by all who heard her brilliant words.

What kinds of important considerations can help to alleviate much of the horror associated with the loss of a loved one in a hopeless situation? Not only is the misery of loss an empty feeling, but also most people are awed by the high technology of contemporary hospitals. Therefore, one initial feeling that the physician can alleviate is the fear of being abandoned. As treatment no longer is possible, many patients worry that their doctors will no longer care for them. Often, as physicians caring for patients with cancer, our relationships with them are long term. As the disease becomes untreatable, maintaining interest can afford an important degree of comfort that drugs cannot possibly provide. If we would all remember this principle, much anxiety and suffering could be eliminated.

More than anything else, patients fear pain. Besides the general debilitation caused by a growing cancer, end-stage malignancy often causes excruciating pain. By making sure that the patient's immediate problems are taken care of **immediately,** the problems of long-term pain management can be addressed intelligently. This commitment to comfort provides a sense of well-being essential to effective care of the terminally ill patient. Along with this commitment to comfort is an awareness of the frame of reference of the dying patient. What difference does it make if the terminally ill yet relatively functional individual becomes a narcotic addict? These patients are not going to get better. We are not concerned about misuse of drugs with potential abuse. We are concerned that a patient with a hopeless disease is comfortable. To that end, a few minutes spent teaching how to use narcotics, either oral or intravenous, can create a responsibility in a patient and family that will provide a new sense of importance and add to the feeling of well-being. These concepts were clarified for me at a lecture by Joy Ufema, a nurse thanatologist. Her contributions to this field have been invaluable to oncologic care.

How many times have you heard someone telling you that the doctor said I had 3 months to live and here I am 2 years later? The converse may also be true. The important issue is it cannot possibly be beneficial to the physician, the patient, or the family to put a time on remaining life.

One of the ways I handle the question of "How much time do I have?" is by saying that I do not like to answer the question because I have as good a chance of being wrong as right. I am glad to discuss averages, but remember that averages only mean what happens to a large population. By taking this approach, the patient and family can have a frame of reference in which to develop a perspective without having to focus on an arbitrary time created by the anecdotal experience of the treating physician.

To conclude, it is worthwhile spending some time discussing the end of life. Most experienced oncologists know when a patient is in the last days of life. Ultimately, patients with incurable illnesses die. Remissions turn to relapses, and treatment failures turn to terminal disease. Nonmalignant complications occur with almost routine frequency. Gentle and understanding explanations of the situation can avoid unnecessary medical treatments that add nothing except needless costs. Many patients obtain documents called Living Wills that direct physicians to withhold life-sustaining treatments in the event their diseases become hopeless. A perfect example is the treatment of infections in the moribund or comatose patient. When a patient or family agrees that enough has been done and it is time to die, it is perfectly appropriate to withhold antibiotics for an established infection or even to stop antibiotics and allow the end to come. This does not mean that careful attention to maintaining comfort while withdrawing life-prolonging measures should not be fastidious. The same applies to blood products. If a patient with terminal illness has a decreasing blood count and needs blood to sustain life, there is no reason to continue unnecessary life-prolonging transfusions.

There comes a point in the care of the terminally ill patient when it clearly is time to die. The patient may decide this himself or herself or, if that is not possible, the patient's family may make the decision. When that time comes, the moral obligation of the physician is to facilitate the event in an acceptable and passive fashion. The term passive emphasizes that active euthanasia is not legal and is vastly different from withholding life-prolonging measures.

I lost a patient who had a preleukemic disease called refractory anemia with excessive blasts and for whom I had been caring for more than 2 years. This condition requires only transfusions for management. This beautiful and intelligent lady was doing magnificently and was resigned to her regular transfusion program. Suddenly, her disease converted to virulent acute leukemia. The progression of the leukemia was rapid, and she could not live long without treatment. Unfortunately, treatment is rarely successful. The patient requested a second opinion at the Johns Hopkins Adult Leukemia Center, which we rapidly granted. Our consensus that treatment was not indicated was corroborated by the physicians at Johns Hopkins. The patient agreed. On her return to Franklin Square, she had a fever, and pneumonia was diagnosed. She asked me to do everything I could to treat her pneumonia and immediately requested that her four children join her from different parts of the United States. We vigorously treated her lung infection, and all four children flew to Baltimore. Her leukemia continued to progress rapidly. After 2 days of going over affairs with her family and saying the words she felt she needed to say, this beautiful and brilliant lady said she had had enough. I was called into her room to hear her say, "Michael, I'm ready to die and would like no more treatment." We stopped her antibiotics, maintained her mouth care and hydration to avoid nausea, discontinued all blood products, prescribed tranquilizers and morphine as necessary to control her discomfort, and thus allowed her to exit peacefully by the next morning. I miss her.

I close by discussing the removal of life support when all hope of recovery is gone. This is a much more difficult decision than not starting life support in the first place. As long as patient, family, and physician agree, it is appropriate, reasonable, and legal to disconnect the respirator, stop administering cardiac drugs to maintain blood pressure, and discontinue antibiotics. There is a time to live and a time to die. Nothing oncologists learn in medical school, residency, or fellowship teaches us when that time is. We do, however, know when a situation is hopeless, and it is the patient's and family's prerogative to make the decision to stop all treatment. As oncologists, it is our moral charge to facilitate such wishes.

Epilog

If the book accomplished only one thing, I hope it emphasized how important clear and understandable information is. Communication between treaters and patients is as important as the treatment itself. Patients can obtain excellent information about oncology and malignant diseases in many ways. The American Cancer Society has a wonderful service that provides pamphlets about most malignancies. You may call them to obtain this information; they are prompt and courteous. The National Cancer Institute has a service that informs patients and their families of new treatment protocols that are available in their areas. This information is more sophisticated but is readily available and often very useful. Most cancer centers have support groups in which patients with cancers discuss their feelings. The one at my center is called "I Can Cope." Many patients take advantage of these organizations and derive a significant amount of comfort and peace. The bottom line is: you are entitled to know. Avail yourselves of your options to get information. Never take "no" for an answer.